ADVANCE PRAISE

"Ashley's story is a masterclass in what happens when belief meets action. In 2010, I supported her run across America because I believed in the power of one voice to make a difference. What she's built since—a nonprofit and movement captured in a compelling and beautifully written memoir—is inspiring. This book is for anyone who's ever asked, 'Can I really do this?' The answer is yes. You are strong enough to do anything."

MONTEL WILLIAMS,
Veteran, MS Advocate, and
Emmy Award Winning Television Host

"I believe that storytelling is one of the most powerful tools we have. It heals, it connects, it galvanizes. *The Long Run Home* will do all of that and more. It reminds us that our hardest moments can become our most profound chapters, and that the road, while long, is also lined with grace."

ROBIN ARZÓN,
VP of Fitness Programming at Peloton,
NYT Best-Selling Author, Ultramarathoner

"Guts, grit, heart. Easy words to say, but few among us put ourselves to such a grueling test as Ashley Schneider has. *The Long Run Home* is a roadmap back to youthful audacity, but told by a wise woman with many miles of successful fundraising and nonprofit leadership to her name. Gorgeously written, this memoir is also a love letter from a daughter to a mother, in the vein of *Refuge* by Terry Tempestt Williams and *Wild* by Cheryl Strayed. Read it if you run. Read it if you don't. Just read it."

AMANDA GERSH,
Author, Editor, Creative Strategist

"Ashley's story is something that stays with you long after you finish the final page. Running across America is impressive in itself, but when you learn about the trials and tribulations of getting from California to New York in an RV, it goes from impressive to unforgettable. When you mix in Ashley's motivation to honor her mother's fight with multiple sclerosis, the book becomes a moving testament to love and the power of purpose. I was hooked on this book from the first page, inspired by Ashley's grit, determination, and love behind every mile. This book is a powerful reminder that we really can do hard things."

TRENNI CASEY,
Sports Anchor and Reporter, NBC Boston

"As an ultrarunner living with MS, I finished this book feeling more resolute, inspired to take on audacious challenges even when the path is unclear. Ashley writes with honesty and vulnerability, opening a window into how MS impacts a family. The miles are real, the heat is punishing, and the love is steady. Her determination sparked MS Run the US and has inspired countless others. This book carries that spark forward, inviting each of us to choose purpose, move with hope, and keep going."

MATT KNAGGS,
RUNNING WITH MS Group Founder,
Keynote Speaker, MS Advocate

The Long Run Home

The Long Run Home

A DAUGHTER'S RUN ACROSS AMERICA
TO FIGHT MS

ASHLEY M. SCHNEIDER

THE LONG RUN HOME
A Daughter's Run Across America to Fight MS

Copyright © 2025 by Ashley M. Schneider

All rights reserved. No part of this book may be reproduced, distributed, or transmitted in any form or by any means, including photocopying, recording, or other electronic or mechanical methods, without the written permission from the publisher or author, except as permitted by U.S. copyright law or in the case of brief quotations embodied in a book review.

Disclaimer: This book has been published for the purpose of providing the reader with general information on its subject matter. The author and the publisher believe the information to be accurate and authoritative at the time of publication. The book is sold with the understanding that neither the author nor the publisher is providing professional advice, and the reader should not rely upon this book as such. Every situation is different, and professional advice (whether psychological, legal, financial, tax, or otherwise) should only be obtained from a professional licensed in your jurisdiction who has knowledge of the specific facts and circumstances.

Interior Layout and Design by Stephanie Anderson
Book Cover Design by Alex Kirkland
Editorial Team: Ginny Glass, Becca Blackburn, and Kiska Carr
Author Headshot Photography by Angela Steenhagen

ISBNs:
979-8-89165-324-5 *Paperback*
979-8-89165-325-2 *Hardback*
979-8-89165-323-8 *E-book*

Published by:
Streamline Books
Kansas City, MO
streamlinebookspublishing.com

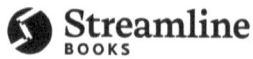

For my family—given and chosen.

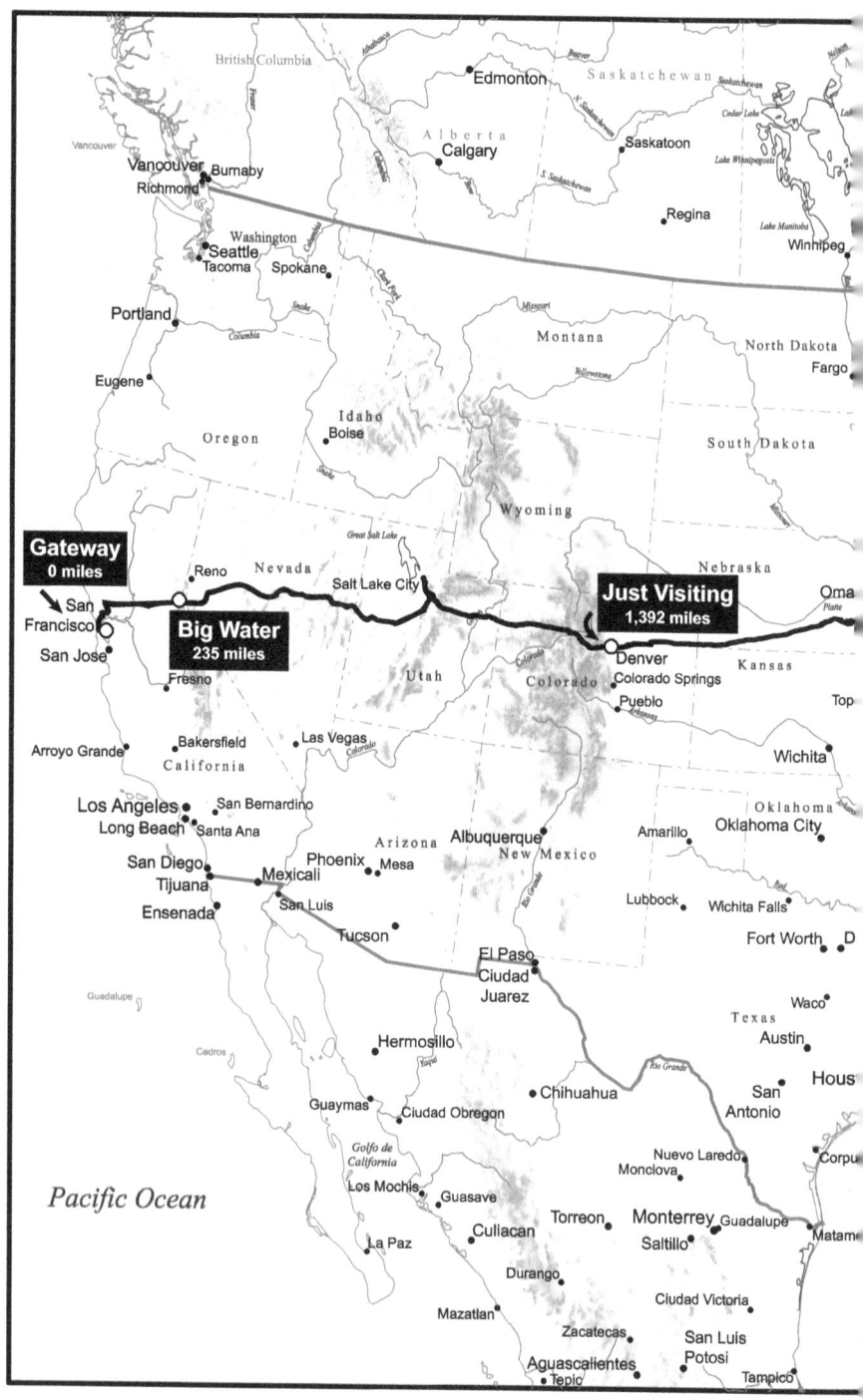

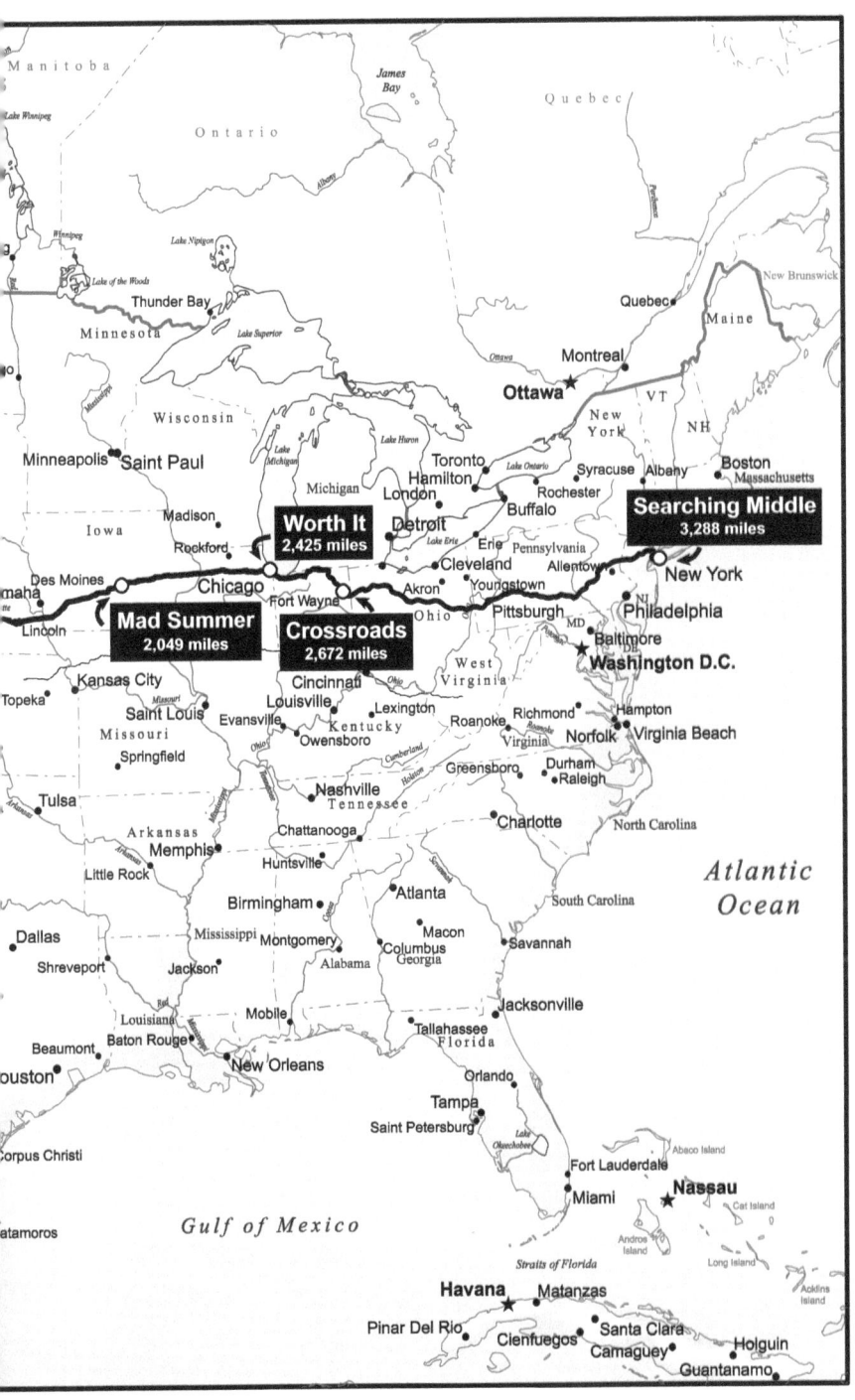

CONTENTS

Foreword . . . . **xi**
Introduction . . . . **xv**

PART 1: LEADING TO THIS

1 Leading to This. **3**
2 Sweat. **9**
3 Then Do It Now. **18**

PART 2: RUNNING HOME

4 The Date Is Set **27**
5 Gateway **42**
6 Tracks **54**
7 Run On **65**
8 Big Water **78**
9 Snowcapped **89**
10 Edges **110**
11 Settled Dust **127**
12 Colorful Colorado. **141**
13 Tough Act to Follow **162**
14 Just Visiting **174**
15 Running Home **189**
16 The Good Life **204**
17 Mad Summer **218**
18 Sloshing **228**
19 Worth It **242**

PART 3: SEARCHING MIDDLE

20 Crossroads **265**
21 Linger **286**
22 Searching Middle **299**

Notes **303**
Acknowledgments **307**
About the Author **309**

FOREWORD

SOME RUNS CHANGE YOU. Others change the world. Ashley Schneider's run across America did both. When I first heard about her journey—thousands of miles, one step at a time, for her mother and everyone affected by multiple sclerosis—it didn't strike me as wild. It struck me as true. When someone you love is living with MS, you learn that healing doesn't always look like stillness. Sometimes it looks like action. Like motion. Like doing the hardest, most beautiful thing you can think of—and then doing it again tomorrow. She inspired me to sign up for my first multiday ultra challenge, MS Run the US, and those runs, five marathons in five days, changed the trajectory of my life.

As an ultramarathoner, I know the road intimately. The early mornings. The aching feet. The silence between steps when the body is screaming and the soul responds, "Keep going." But Ashley's story isn't just about miles logged or muscles pushed to their edge. It's about love. And grief. And healing. And the radical choice to take pain—hers, her mother's, her family's—and alchemize it into purpose.

This book, *The Long Run Home*, is a portrait of grit. Not the hashtag kind. The real kind. The kind you develop when you watch someone you love—in Ashley's case, her mother—slowly lose parts of themselves to a disease that never asks permission. My mother also lives with multiple sclerosis, and I run for her. So yes, this story is deeply personal to me too. It's the story of my mother's strength. Our family's resilience. It's the story of every mile I've run to reclaim agency in the face of something that tries to steal it.

As mothers, we hold our families with arms and hearts stretched wide. As athletes, we often channel our emotions through movement. And as women, we know what it means to carry more than our share—sometimes with grace, sometimes with gritted teeth. Ashley's journey speaks to all of this.

When she left behind a life of adventure working on cruise ships to run 3,288 miles across the country, she wasn't doing it for fame, or finish lines, or sponsorship deals. She did it because something inside her said, "This is the way. This is how you show up for your people." That kind of clarity doesn't come easy. It's forged through years of pain and perspective—of watching her mom lose one small ability at a time, and deciding that grief wouldn't be the end of the story.

Ashley ran to reconnect with herself, to reclaim what MS had stolen from her family, and to raise awareness for a disease that still needs more voices, more advocacy, and more action. What she created—a national nonprofit, a legacy run, and a storytelling movement—is proof that the road you choose can change the world, if you're bold enough to step into it.

This isn't just a memoir. It's a manifesto of resilience. It's about learning how to take the long way home—back to your truth, back to your roots, back to the people who shaped you.

If you are an athlete, you will feel the heartbeat of every training day etched into these pages. If you are a caregiver or a child of someone living with chronic illness, you will find comfort in knowing you are not alone. If you are someone who's ever wondered, *Can I really do this?* let this book answer you: Yes. You can. One step at a time.

Ashley's honesty in sharing the messiness—not just the finish line moments—is what makes this book special. She writes about the detours, the fears, the physical and emotional toll. She writes about the days when she didn't want to lace up, and the moments she found meaning in unexpected places—a stranger's generosity,

FOREWORD

a stretch of open highway, a call from someone just needing to feel seen.

I believe that storytelling is one of the most powerful tools we have. It heals, it connects, it galvanizes. *The Long Run Home* will do all of that and more. It reminds us that our hardest moments can become our most profound chapters, and that the road, while long, is also lined with grace.

To anyone reading this who is navigating your own version of the long run—whether it's motherhood, illness, recovery, or just the weight of being human—know this: You're not alone. And if you ever forget how strong you are, let Ashley's words light a spark. We've got miles to cover. And we're not alone.

—Robin Arzón

INTRODUCTION

MANY YEARS HAVE PASSED since I ran across America for my mother—to take a stand against multiple sclerosis (MS) and how it battered my life. Much has changed since then—both around me and within me. I often think of who I was at the beginning of this story—how I couldn't have possibly imagined what was to come or how much good could be created from a simple, whole-hearted yes.

If I had known, I believe I would have been overwhelmed. But I'm deeply grateful for being brave enough to start—despite the absurdity of the idea—to see what might become of it.

It is my deepest desire that, in my story, you find the bravery to say yes to the wild, good-natured ideas that cross your mind—the ones that don't quite make sense, yet stir something in you; the ones that grip you and refuse to let go.

I share the story of my run across America as a witness—to the unfolding, and to the community that swelled in the wake of that journey.

To write this book, I drew from my personal journals, blog posts, social media updates, photo albums, and notes about the route, people, places, and events I encountered. I have changed the names of many—though not all—individuals, and in some cases, altered identifying details to protect their privacy. There are no composite characters or fabricated events in this book. Some moments and experiences were left out, but only if they did not impact the heart or message of the story.

PART 1
Leading to This

"Champions aren't born, they create themselves through hard, sweat-filled work. They dazzle us with their talent and make us believe anything is possible." -UNKNOWN

CHAPTER ONE

Leading to This

A LOT CAN HAPPEN in three miles.

I'd discover that soon enough as my harpsichord alarm awoke me from my slumber. The melody chimed from my phone, and in the complete darkness of a room with no windows, I quieted the sound and crept out of my bunk. The floor of the ship rocked ever so slightly as it sailed into port. My roommate would sleep later, so I slipped into the bathroom, a tight space four feet wide and four feet long, and flipped on a fluorescent light that beamed above the mirror. I was up before dawn, as I often was, to exercise and shake out the drinks from the night before. I took inventory of my face—smudged mascara and some puffiness, but not too bad. I turned on the hot water and washed it all away.

Once dressed in cotton shorts, a sports bra, a gray *Orthopedic Sports Medicine* T-shirt, and running shoes, I pulled my pixie cut hair into spike pigtails and brushed my teeth. I was on the second deck of the ship, located in the hull—as low as one could go without dropping into the engine rooms and cargo spaces. This is where the crew slept.

The ship I was working on was on a two-week repeat tour of Europe at the tail end of the summer season, churning waters from England to Spain, to Italy, to Africa, and then back again.

I'd boarded my first cruise ship two years prior, a used and outdated one doing weekend trips from Los Angeles, and since then, I had smiled my way up to the newest ship in the fleet. As sports staff, I helped manage the activity deck with a close-knit group of coworkers. It was a coveted position, our workspace being on the top deck of the ship in the open air, 230 feet above the water. We had a panoramic view of the ocean, and it was the only staff position that didn't work when it rained.

When I clocked in, I did things like belay a forty-foot rock wall and teach passengers how to surf on our simulated wave machine. I layered on sunblock but still tanned like a Texas cowboy, my slathering being no match to the hours I spent breathing in the salty sea air. When in port, the sports deck closed down to push the passengers off the boat, and I got to do the same. "What'd you think?" we'd ask each other, "Should we head into Rome or go to that winery instead?" I went shopping in London and lay on the beaches of Nice. I toured the French Riviera by helicopter and ate authentic Italian pizza *in* Italy. I surfed the streets of Portugal (quite literally on a wooden sled) and marveled at the Colosseum. I visited Rome, the Rock of Gibraltar, the Canary Islands, Ireland.

People ask why, at the age of twenty-four, having never run a marathon before, I quit this dream job of mine to run 125 consecutive marathons across America; why, with zero fundraising experience, I decided to raise half a million dollars for multiple sclerosis. I write it out in a single sentence, and it all sounds so absurd. Especially when there were other, more ill-fitting factors, like the fact that I stumbled tipsy to bed many nights a week, loved to travel and was being paid to do it, relished a good joint on the beach, and had no intentions of doing anything different for the foreseeable future. I wasn't looking for a reason to rectify the pain I carried from my mother's disease with a pair of running shoes. I was looking for a free drink at the bar and what connections I needed to get a contract through Alaska.

There is no simple answer except to say that, over the course of a three-mile run in Barcelona, it came to me that everything that had happened in my life led to this—that it had been waiting for me to come upon it all along. And for reasons that I still wonder about today, I trusted it.

I was twenty-two years old when I boarded my first ship, and I didn't look back for exactly twenty-five months and twenty-three days when I found reason to believe that the thing that drove me there would actually be the thing to bring me home. It was called multiple sclerosis, and it battered my life. Like raging waters beating on an earthen shore, it eroded pieces of my mother away one affliction at a time until most of what remained were the lessons that I learned in its presence. That and her essence, which elegantly withstood the storms.

She loved bacon and Jesus, not equally but almost, and watched *Young and the Restless* every day at 11:00 a.m. on CBS 58. Her breath smelled of sweet cinnamon gum, and she was the kind of lady who wore pantyhose with both her dresses and pants. Standing at five foot nothing, she towered in a crowd, beaming with joy so abundant her eyes smiled even when no one was looking—people gravitated toward her because of it. An optimist and an extrovert, she had a true interest in people and also loved them.

"It happened again." My dad would chuckle. "I sat her on the bench outside the doctor's office, and by the time I got back, she had a new best friend. 'See ya later, Nancy!' I heard her say. What a piece of work."

She beamed at his side, grinning while he recalled the story.

She was my mother and what I knew a woman to be, so when parts of her began disappearing, I grieved their departure like a deep loss—portions of her that I adored drifting away in the storm.

I was eight when we gave up biking—her leaving the house with me riding at her side, her skidding into a ditch after losing her balance, and us walking back together—her bruised and bloody. At eleven, it was waterskiing—her trying relentlessly to "pop out of the water" as she always had, us watching from the speed boat, cheering her on, her becoming so fatigued that my father had to pull her from the water. At fourteen, I listened from the steps while her hands fumbled along the piano keys, trying to find that once-graceful melody. It was gone.

By the time I sailed upon the seas, she had endured a thousand losses, and my concept of what a mother should be—helpful, capable, a caregiver—had died a thousand times too. My mom. Jill. Jillebean. Tiny and loving, everyone adored her, especially my father.

I came along third in their line of wild offspring. Marriage. My sister, April. Multiple sclerosis. Aaron. Ashley. Dawn—all born just a few years apart. "D for done," Mom would say after rattling off our names. She always had a cutesy way of spelling things out. "K-U-M as in merry-L-I-E-N as in nice" was our last name.

They met in a bar in Milwaukee. My father was the audio tech for a band, and my mother was a catching young blonde who came to a show. She lingered some time after the set, drinking a white zinfandel and sending glances his way—a handsome fella with shaggy brown hair and a chevron mustache. She wasn't bad to look at, he thought, and much to his surprise, her beauty wasn't only skin deep. She listened intently with delighted eyes and touched his arm just so when he told a joke, throwing her head back in a laugh.

"Would you like another glass?" he asked.

She said, "Thank you," with blushing cheeks. If he had asked her to marry him then, I imagine she would have said yes, being the romantic that she was, but my father was a procrastinator. The proposal materialized years later, only at the possibility of losing her. Five years of courtship and no ring, Jill walked away from the relationship, leaving Keith right where she found him, with his buddies in a bar.

"I sat on that bar stool looking around, wondering what the hell was my problem," he'd say later, telling the story. "I was never going to find a better gal than your mother." Keith left the bar that night and went straight to Jill's apartment, banging on her door at two in the morning. "She opened the door, and I said, 'All right. We'll get married, but we're going to have a long engagement.'"

Six months later, they tied the knot. Jill had a tender way of getting her way.

Dawn was a blessing surprise that came after my parents decided three kids were enough. "I'd have as many as we could make

LEADING TO THIS

if it had been up to me," Dad would say. What he meant was that multiple sclerosis put a timeline on their family planning.

The disease is unpredictable that way, attacking anyone at any time and being completely unique in its progression. One could manage mild symptoms for the rest of their life or end up in a wheelchair by the end of the year. The majority of those diagnosed fluctuate somewhere between those two, but the worst-case scenario is terrifying. My mother lay still during her first MRI scan as best she could and hoped for a simple answer to the unexplainable sickness she felt—nausea, headaches, and dizziness for days on end. She thought it was the flu, but when it didn't go away, they scanned her brain.

"Are you claustrophobic?" the machine tech asked. She shook her head no. "Do you have anything metallic in you? A heart stint? Pacemaker? Any pumps or surgeries of any sort?"

She was almost sure no, but now she wondered, Did she? Could something have happened when she was younger and wasn't told? No, no, there was nothing, she was sure. She shook her head no.

"Do you have anything in your pockets? In your hair? Buckles or fasteners of any sort? It's very important you have no metal objects in you or on you."

The questioning made her nervous. Her husband stood in the waiting room, soothing their eighteen-month-old child. What if she was wrong? What if there was something? No, no, she had it right. There was nothing. She shook her head no.

The results came back, and what her family got was an answer of complex unknowns in the form of a degenerative disease they had never heard of—multiple sclerosis. The Greek name meant *many scars*, and the disease coursed through her central nervous system, wreaking havoc on the pathways between the brain and the body. It was 1980, and science was only just beginning its research.

With my father gone during the day at work, they took a gamble, having three more kids, not knowing if, when, or how severely her health might decline. Who would take care of us kids *and* our mother? How would they make it work? It was a belief in something higher—a trust in their path despite these challenging circumstances. Too much good to measure has come from that willingness.

Later, when I heard these stories, I wondered if the many scars were just hers or if they included the ones we endured as a family. Pain, numbness, fatigue, and mental fog were a few of her regular symptoms. But the more troublesome ones, like immobility and bladder dysfunction, appeared and lingered at the most inconvenient times.

I was fourteen when things turned bad.

CHAPTER TWO

Sweat

"**YOU'RE BEING A SELFISH BITCH!**" my brother screamed at me in my bedroom, standing inches from my face. "Go see Mom!"

"I have a math test on Friday and a cross-country meet on Saturday. What do you want me to do?" I shouted back. "Fail math?"

"Fuck math!" He seethed. "You know better."

I did know better, but, *God*, I didn't want to see her that way. It had been seventeen days since Dawn found her rigid as a board, convulsing in a seizure, and slumped off the couch in front of *The Oprah Winfrey Show*. We were at school. Dad was at work. I went to cross-country practice after my final class of the day and missed the caravan to the hospital, where they would tell my father that she had been seizing for hours and now her brain was fried. I ran, my brother got angry, Dawn wouldn't leave her side, and April rebelled. We were all navigating what happened the best we could at the ages of eighteen, sixteen, fourteen, and ten—but damage had been done all around.

The seizure wasn't technically a symptom of her MS, but it also didn't exactly mean it wasn't—her nervous system was a wreck, and the scars along her brain and spinal cord didn't help the recovery one bit. They set her up in an inpatient rehabilitation bed, and

I found every excuse not to witness her relearning how to walk, write, and bring yogurt to her face with a spoon.

"What'd ya think, kid?" my father would ask, picking me up from cross-country practice.

"I'm really hungry," I'd say. "We did hill repeats all hour. Can we go home first so I can eat?"

"We can grab something on the way?" he'd say, pulling out of the high school parking lot.

"I know. I've gotta shower too. And do homework. I'm all sweaty."

"Yeah, okay," he'd reply. He was never one to press.

But my brother wasn't my father, at least not in this way, and he called out my bullshit until I said I would go. I arrived at the hospital the next day as they helped her eat—she was propped up by pillows in a hospital bed, controlling her spoon like a baby. I pulled up a chair and put my palm over her free hand, still on her lap. She smiled at me and gurgled a few sounds, attempting to speak. I caught the word *missed*.

"I missed you too," I whispered, and I always would from that moment on. She never would fully regain her function.

"How about a shower when you're done?" I asked. Her hair was messy and matted down, the way it gets when one lies in bed for days and is cleaned by sponge baths.

Lathering her head in the handicapped shower stall, I held my breath, overwhelmed by the smell of the hospital corridors—all that neediness. All that sterile, sick air.

Years later, I would think of this moment in college after landing a job at an inpatient physical therapy unit at the hospital downtown—a cushy, well-paying job that lined my resume for the doctorate program I sought. I would hold puke buckets for strangers and rub the backs of other people's mothers. *See*, I'd reason with God, *I'm compassionate. I've changed. I'd take care of Mom if she weren't hours away.*

I offered these things and meant them, not knowing how God would test me on my promises.

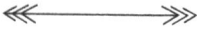

SWEAT

I HIT QUICK START, and the treadmill hummed to life in the state-of-the-art fitness center on the ship. Located on the fourteenth floor, the room had floor-to-ceiling windows at the front facing the ocean. The running machines lined up in a neat row there, where my reflection on the glass bounced back at me from the darkened morning sky. Beyond it, beyond the low, lapping waves, the Barcelona city lights illuminated a sleepy harbor like a string of café lights pulled across the earth. The belt I stood upon inched into motion at first, then gained speed. And with it too, I hummed to life.

Mile one.

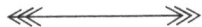

"OKAY, IT'S TIME TO pick your events." The gym teacher called out, "One track and two field, or two track and one field, but you have to pick one of each."

I was in first grade at the same private, K-through-eighth-grade Lutheran school my mother had attended, and we were selecting events for my favorite week of the year—track and field.

The pop gun would sound, and I'd take off with a line of kids from my class to test myself along the painted lines marking the track on the elementary school parking lot. I pumped my arms and cycled my legs as fast as I could—feeling the rush and feeling free. In between events, I'd sit on a patch of lawn with my friends, eating an apple with the sun shining on my face, watching the other children. It was heaven, and it was home.

I always chose the same three events—the four-hundred- and eight-hundred-meter races (the longest ones available) and running long jump. After the week was over, I would stand in my bedroom staring at the three ribbons I'd earned. They were satin pieces of cloth with gold etching, all the same royal-blue color. *First Place.*

Winning was exciting, but even into high school, where I experienced true competition and defeats, I loved it. At the time, like many teens, I felt reservations about wholly being myself. I graduated from that private elementary school with a class of thirty-six students and was thrown into a public school the next district over. None of my childhood friends would be with me.

"It'll be good for you," my parents said, "We can't send you to private high school, so it is what it is."

I hated it—arriving to the wide halls and tall ceilings, stuffing my things into a locker and walking to class alone, sitting next to whoever in class, not knowing if they were cool or not cool and if talking to them would be social suicide, not knowing where or *if* I fit in. A tight ball formed in my stomach, and the only place it unraveled was at cross-country practice.

"Okay, we've got an easy mile warm-up to the park, and I mean *easy*, ladies. And then we've got a set of seven two-hundred-meter repeats in the grass," Coach John bellowed, looking over his clipboard. "Once we're there, I'll show you the start and finish and shout out your pace times."

As soon as he gave us the go, we'd run off, laughing.

This, I could do. I knew exactly how I measured up. Did I warm up well? Did I hit my paces? Was I feeling off, and if yes, why? Did I crush it, and if yes, why? I ate well, I never drank soda, and Coach taught us the value of sleep for recovery. Before meets, he'd take us to a classroom and dim the lights.

"Okay, lie on your backs, close your eyes, and put your hands on your belly to feel your breath."

We did as he said. Then he'd talk us through a visualization of the course and how we would run it. Sure, he was a little odd, and this was a little weird, but what about my life wasn't a bit of both at this point? Everything was a mess, and I appreciated the opportunity he gave me to envision my best possible future.

Then my mother ended up in the hospital for over a month, and I ran.

"What'd you guys do after the Poms competition on Saturday?" one popular girl asked the other during class. I sat nearby, pretending not to listen.

"My mom took me shopping and then to lunch. I got an amazing pair of jeans. My butt looks so good in them. I'll show you after school."

Her mom took her shopping—how perfect. What could I even add to this conversation? "Hey, cool. I gave my mom a shower, and then I sat by while the occupational therapist taught her how to stack blocks on a spindle."

I didn't want to talk about it, but I also couldn't think about much else either. Social anxiety wedged itself in my mind—a distance between them and me that flourished under my inability to surface from the depths of what was happening. It was a precarious, difficult time, and sweat saved me from all the other places a teen has to put anxiety.

Each day, I set out to see how far, hard, and fast I could go—these were things I could control. I lifted weights and showed up for agility practice. I squatted and broad jumped. I crunched and sprinted. I drenched my shirts through to "Smells Like Teen Spirit" blasting so loud that no other thought could break through.

And it wasn't lost on me that every run, every effort, every pound I plated on the bar was a gift. *You get to do this*, I reminded myself. There was no amount of miles I could run that matched the suffering of what life looked like without the option to.

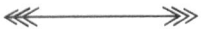

DROP YOUR ARMS. BREATHE. I coached myself on the ship's treadmill. The minutes accumulated on the display, but I had covered that with a gym towel. The minutes wouldn't own me. I owned them by focusing on what I could control—concentrating inward, doing a continuous head-to-toe assessment of form. *Lean forward,* and now gravity was in my favor. *Loosen your shoulders*, and my lungs opened. *Hit the forefoot*, and my stride lightened. The belt of the treadmill whipped below me, and I ran. Everything was about what my body was doing and whatever thoughts emerged.

Today's tour in Barcelona is going to be awesome! La Sagrada Familia and Casa Milà. I can't wait to tell Steph about Camp Nou. So cool. I wonder what time the gangway opens tomorrow. I'd love to run here before we leave. I can't believe how much I've seen of Europe.

I was two years old when I caught a knack for exploring. Mile two.

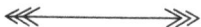

"DO YOU KNOW WHERE Ashley is?" Grandma questioned my mother over the phone.

Looking over her shoulder curiously, my mother searched for her third-born among the clothes and clutter that crowded the landscape of our living room.

"You can't possibly know because I'm looking at her half-naked self right now."

It wasn't so much that my mother lost her child as it was that I decided to see Grandma and needed no one's permission to do it. I was nearly two and had wandered three blocks to her house just up the street from ours, wearing a onesie and socks. From there, the distances and decisiveness only grew.

"This one's a self-starter," my father would say of me aloud to the neighbors, the grocery store clerk, my coach. I loved his assessment of me, but never thought to apply it to a career, even after a college placement test told me to do so.

"An entrepreneur! Organizational skills!" my father exclaimed while he read the results in our kitchen. "Are you going to own a business like your old man?"

"Hardly." I scoffed. "Nine to five, with benefits. I'm getting a job I can leave behind when I clock out." I had been raised helping the family business—management of a cluster of townhomes my parents bought up from her parents. I knew what that work was like, and I wasn't interested. It was instability. It was stress. It wasn't a job; it was a lifestyle.

"The red house has new tenants moving in next week," my father would say. "I need to get it cleaned up by Saturday, and I could use your help."

I'd march over to the house in a pair of paint-splattered shorts with my siblings, earning ten dollars an hour to rip up carpet, pull nails, varnish floors, scrape the trim, scrub tile, and paint. We'd mow acres of grass, pull shoots of weeds more plentiful than the flowers, and prune row after row of hedges. My father was a truck driver, but he quit when I was a toddler to do this, motivated to provide not only for his family of six but also for a future that might include a long list of expensive medical needs. At times, it even caused them.

I was sixteen when he rushed me to the ER. "Where were your gloves?" he pressed, driving with a hurried focus. I held a dish towel to my trembling hand, staring in hot pain at all the blood, furious at myself for being so self-assured, for learning my own way. If I were to be in the sun for four hours straight, I would have a great tan to show for it, I decided, tossing the leather work gloves down on the toolbox. Dad worries too much; nothing bad is going to happen. I grabbed the electric trimmer and hacked at the bushes, then nearly severed two fingers.

It wasn't the labor that deterred me—even after lopping my hand. I enjoyed the hard work and sweat. It was security that I craved, and starting my own business was hardly that.

My father was doing the best he could, but his plate was full. Full full—a handicapped wife, four children, twelve rental units (with their leaky faucets, broken heaters, and clogged toilets at all hours), bills, sports tournaments, school activities, grocery shopping, cooking. And all the laundry? My father did it all except the cleaning.

He had a work ethic like no one I knew, but the place things went was whatever surface was in front of him. My mother tried to help where she could, crawling across the floor on all fours, unsteady on her feet but determined, trying to pick this thing up over here and that thing up over there. Growing up, we helped too.

But grown now and off to college, I came back to old newspapers, used dishes, medical syringes, junk mail, dirty clothes, and more pieces of broken furniture than one could possibly repair. No amount of crawling by my mother could undo it.

"Dad, you can't live like this. It's not safe for Mom," I'd preach to him over winter break. "There's no place to walk. She could trip, split her head open. You need some help. You need a maid. Look at this end table. Why are you keeping it?"

"I'm going to fix it," he'd say.
"Dad, when? You have no time."
"Ashley, a man's gotta have his dreams."

Dreams? I'd fume. *Who keeps garbage as dreams?* I longed to get away from it all, so I'd lace up my shoes and run until my lungs screamed.

My father, though, this was his life. He couldn't get away. And truthfully, he cherished my mother, so he never would even if he had the option to. The ways *he* protected himself against the shit of MS were with actual walls made of junk and generous pours of vodka. Stress gathered inside him until it spilled into piles of crap as tall as me and empty handles of Fleischman's strewn about. It hadn't always been that bad, but over time, it became that way. His hoarding and drinking increased along with her disease progression—as Mom's disabilities mounted, so did the things he found to drown in.

I couldn't blame him. It was quite effective.

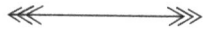

"CHUG! CHUG! CHUG!" THE crowd chanted. I was down on one knee, head-to-head in a Natty Light beer bong race.

"Yeah!" they erupted with the winner. Not me, but I didn't care, diving headfirst into a destructive, binge-drinking habit in college to *finally* fit in. High fives for everyone, jokes all around. The goal wasn't to win. It was to get drunk as fuck. Done. I was a freshman on the university soccer team and a virgin to everything—a church-going daughter of a Jesus-lovin' family that had had no sex, no alcohol, and no drugs in my past, which also meant I had no peers. This had been my life in high school, but now, instead of watching movies with my family on the weekends, I watched them on my own. And I saw what following the rules got a person, witnessing the deterioration of my mother.

Off on my own in college—one church service later, with only hurried hellos and eight weeks of exercising alone at the recreation center, and I was ready to see what else life had to offer.

Screw this, I thought. *Time for some fun.*

I met the girls on my soccer team out at parties with zero experience to guide me and checked off each of those church-going "noes" within a month's time. By "self-starter," my father also meant I didn't throttle much. Everything was full on, including this. Three years later, it would land me in a hospital bed, getting my stomach pumped of poison and a hefty bill to send my parents, but that hardly changed anything. It was a mistake, I told others. Just that one time. It was the hundred-proof shots of SoCo and Coach's fault for enforcing a dry preseason. Can you believe she wants me to get counseling? What a joke. She can't tell me what to do. I don't have a problem. I know my limits.

But I never did.

Drunk, there was no social anxiety, no mangled family, and no unfair God who grants some miracles but not others. I could be anyone, and I was—Samantha and Carmen were my names, and I'd dish them out with a random number, then laugh about it with my girlfriends. There were blurred lines and lots of puke, but even that was more tolerable than all the rest of it.

The only person who knew all these parts of me was Steph, the soccer team's goalie. Like me, from afar, her life looked solid, normal. An athlete with great grades, she was good at hiding as well. It was in hushed tones on the bus rides to games she told me secrets about herself that made me feel safe. She knew what it was like to ache for something better, to watch her family become wrecked by disease while drifting among the perfect lives of everyone else. Her friendship meant so much to me that I gave us a try one drunken night after the football player ended things, only to awaken to a hangover and the affirmation that I desired men. Instead, I would escape to Colorado. There, I could leave these broken shards behind and build a shiny new life in the mountains.

CHAPTER THREE

Then Do It Now

"**SHE NEEDS WIDE OPEN** spaces! Room to make her big mistakes. She needs new faces! She knows the high stakes!" I sang along with the Dixie Chicks blaring through my VW Jetta speakers. I was in my last semester of college, twenty-one years old, and driving west in mid-January across the snowy, wind-whipped plains of Nebraska to my new home–Boulder, Colorado. I was doing it. I was doing it! If not after a bit of effort.

"I'll take out four credit cards if I have to!" I screamed at my father through my phone, "You can't stop me!" Then I slammed the phone shut and hurled it at my mattress. It landed with a *thwack* in a fluff of pillows.

For the first time in my life that I could recall, my father had told me no. "You can't afford it," he had said in a stern voice. My plan was to pass on a well-paid internship in Wisconsin and head to Colorado for an unpaid one. He disagreed.

"Boulder?" he said. "The rent will be four times as much, and you won't be earning any money. That doesn't make sense."

But I hadn't called to ask. I worked part-time as a waitress at the Olive Garden in my college town and would transfer to the one located in Boulder. That money would sustain me–the rent, the food, the bills, all of it. I packed my four-door sedan to the ceiling with everything I owned and hugged my family goodbye on the uneven, gray sidewalk outside my college duplex—a worn and cracked powder-blue home on the north edge of campus. My sister, Dawn, sobbed alongside my mother. He stood beside them sullen, with his hands in his pockets, unable to stop me. I was his third-born but the first to leave. He wasn't taking it well.

And then I saw what he meant.

I counted the money I earned my first week in Boulder and swore under my breath. *Fuck*. The week's tips totaled seventy-five dollars—half of what I would earn per night in Wisconsin. My monthly rent alone was six times that amount. Boulder was an affluent community. Where was everyone eating?

"They're not coming here," a coworker told me. "They're going to Pearl Street."

So that's where I went too—up and down Pearl Street, a boho pedestrian walkway lined with boutique shops and fine dining, handing out my resume. One manager stood next to a chic bar in a French restaurant and asked, "What's face-paced?" pointing out a spelling error on the paper I handed him.

"Oh." I shrugged. "Just a typo. It's supposed to say fast-paced."

He stared at me for a moment, sizing me up. I smiled big.

"Okay, I'll give you a shot," he said. "You start next week. We're opening a new place in North Boulder. You'll work there."

I practically jumped into his arms. "Thank you!"

"Hey," he called after me on my way out. I turned to look at him. "It's kind of a big deal. Don't mess it up."

It was, and I didn't. The new place was a rustic Italian trattoria serving authentic Italian food. The recipes were gathered from actual trips to Italy and cooked by trained chefs who took their craft seriously. The wine was hand-selected by a sommelier, a certified wine specialist, and was poured into hand-blown, seamless glasses.

"Do. Not. Break. These," David instructed the group of servers. "They cost forty-five dollars apiece, and I'll be pissed if you break one."

There were rows of them. *Think of all that money on* glassware, I thought.

But I didn't have to think of it. After that, my own money started pouring in. That job was bank, and I learned quickly that the path that got me started didn't have to be the one that made it work. Even that it was better that way.

Boulder was more than I imagined it would be. The mountains fed my nature-loving, wanderlust soul, and I drew life from an overflowing well of joyful independence and outdoorsy bliss. Even, no doubt, I felt closer to God—mile high and less angry at everything that had been thrown at my family. A thousand miles of separation does wonders for one's ability to ignore what's still going on. I would have stayed there, basking in the wonders of this shiny new life, had something more tempting not spurred me along.

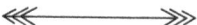

"**DO YOU WANT THE** good news first or the good news first?" I asked my father when he picked up the phone.

"Give me the good news," he replied, playing along.

I had a decision to make.

"I got into doctorate school in Denver," I said. "They bumped up my application after the interview. They want me in the next graduating class."

"Yes! Of course, they did!" He beamed. "Great job, kid. And?"

"Well, Royal Caribbean wants me as well. They can't guarantee a contract now and what ship I'd go on, but I'm in line for the next opening if I want it. So, I don't know. Do I wait for a ship? Or do I head to grad school?"

He exhaled. *Exactly*, I thought. I had worked hard to get into a doctorate PT program—a competitive track that included multiple interviews, essays, applications, and luck. Forty-five applicants were accepted in each class out of hundreds. To pass on the opportunity meant doing the process all over again when I wanted another chance.

He listened patiently while I weighed my options. He always was a good listener—speaking only when necessary or after a few cocktails.

THEN DO IT NOW

I could picture him now on the other end of the line, wearing his favorite camouflage pants and smelling of Old Spice after a clean shave, his face bare except for his chevron mustache. The phone was resting on one ear with his arm draped over the top of his head, muting the noise from the other side. This was a posture he adopted after a raging fever decades prior had nearly taken his life. Instead, it just took the hearing in his left ear.

My mother saved him, the story went. "I'll quit smoking if you let him live," she prayed, bartering with God at my father's bedside in the hospital. As a stay-at-home mother with four kids who was losing the love of her life, she needed to barter—his fever mounting, the doctors losing hope, her being the devoted, praying type. And it worked. He lived, less his hearing, and she never touched a cigarette again.

"You know, Meister," said my father through the phone, using his pet name for me and finally offering his advice, "Your mom and I started a family right away. We wanted to travel after you kids were grown, but it's different now." He went quiet with emotion, then cleared his throat. "Listen. You never know what's going to happen. You're young. You're healthy. If you have the opportunity to do something like travel, then do it now."

His support was a change from the fight we had months prior during my move out west, but I didn't press. It likely had to do with all the ways in which the move challenged me—hustling for a new job, managing a hit and run on my car, fully accepting every bill as mine—and how I rose to these occasions. I stood taller because of them. And now, with his blessing, I was affirmed in what I already felt to be true.

The world was waiting, and I would go after it.

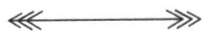

I'VE SEEN SO MUCH of Europe on foot. I wonder what it would be like to see the United States the same way. Where would I go?

The thoughts continued to flow on the treadmill. I watched the port authorities stroll along the Barcelona pier, preparing for the ship to dock. *The Redwoods in California would be amazing. Denver, obviously. And, really, they're not that far apart, right? I wonder how long it'd take to run between the two? Maybe a month? I could run for a month.*

Fueled by endorphins, doing that seemed manageable. I felt agile and light—my mind, distorted in athletic flow. I had never run more than two hours at one time, so I couldn't reason what running for five hours every day for thirty days would be like. But in the moment, it was just a thought, just something to think about.

Has anyone ever done that? Run from California to Colorado? That would be so cool. I wonder how many miles it is. It can't be that far. I bet it's the same as Colorado to Wisconsin, and I've driven that how many times? I could definitely run that distance. Actually...

Thinking about the sixteen-hour road trips I spent in my car driving between the two states, I imagined myself running along the highway instead. Doable.

I should! How cool would it be to run from Colorado to Wisconsin? Home to home! And if I'm going that far, why stop? I could run the whole thing! Has anyone ever done that? Run across America? How many miles is that? How would I even do that?

My mind took off, generating a plan of how I'd manage twenty miles a day in four increments—running for an hour, then taking a break, running for another hour, then taking another break. It seemed simple when I reasoned I'd have nothing else to do except eat, run, and sleep.

What would Mom and Dad say?

The thought of my parents made something click.

Shit.

Mom.

I should do it for Mom.

Holy shit.

Mile three.

I powered down the treadmill and stood still, thinking about it—run across America for my mother. Like, *literally* run across America.

I wanted nothing more than for my mom to be healthy and for

us to be a regular family. To not have a mother who couldn't care for herself, much less me. But that didn't happen, and so I ran. I ran to forget myself. I ran to forget her multiple sclerosis. My whole life, I ran to get away.

Until now.

Walking toward the gym exit, I grabbed a towel and wiped the sweat from my face. The idea was ridiculous and massive, and by outward standards, I lacked the experience to do it. But it was in me, and I knew it. I need only dig it out.

I pushed the heavy gym door open and descended a steel staircase to my crew cabin. I was on the ship still, but I was already gone.

PART 2

Running Home

CHAPTER FOUR

The Date Is Set

BY THE TIME I arrived at the Golden Gate Bridge in San Francisco to begin my 3,288-mile run across America, seventeen months had gone by since the idea had come to me in Barcelona, and I had done all the absurd and impossible things I needed to do to prepare for such a thing. I quit my job with the cruise ship company and moved back into my parents' junk-filled home. I ran a marathon, finally, and then countless more to prepare my body. I built a website for the event and founded a charity. I was given a motorhome and then sponsorship. I was outfitted with clothes, gear, shoes, and more supplies than I knew what to do with.

Most importantly, though, I had support. Not just the kind one gets from family and friends, but real in-person help from the driver who would shuttle me to and from the route every day. He would be at my side, guiding and protecting me. He'd assist me with all the things that needed to be done besides the running—like moving camp, loading gear, shopping, cooking, cleaning, and more. Much more. He would be with me through the high highs and low lows of running five hours nearly every day for six months straight, from one city to the next, across an entire continent.

His name was Nate, and he was from Australia. He was my boyfriend and as new to me as the endeavor itself.

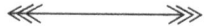

"THEY WORK IN THE casino," my girlfriend shouted into my ear over the roar of the ship's propellers. Music thumped from the ceiling speakers in an attempt to drown it out. We stood at the crew bar located on the lower deck near the back of the ship, ordering drinks.

"Do you know any of them?" I shouted back, looking at a group of three guys standing at a table.

"Only the taller one with the gelled hair. He was sleeping with one of the spa girls on my last ship. His friend's name is Nate. I know that because Liza called dibs when we picked up the ship in Norway."

"And?" I asked. I didn't know Liza. She had no dibs on me. "She get anywhere?"

"Not that I know of," she answered, reaching for her drink. "Let's say hi."

Nate was handsome. Sensual, full lips and a firm jaw shaded just so. Midnight brows above milk chocolate eyes. Athletic and an Aussie, Nate's look was both rugged and groomed. His shoulders were hard with muscle, and his accent was velvety smooth. He smelled of salty sea air with hints of mandarin and sage—a familiar, cozy beach on a flawless summer day. What made him irresistible, though, were his other qualities—his sensitivities, his loyalty, his touch. He'd tear up at the most unexpected times, like when he recalled home, and despite years of travel, he still remained close with each of his friends.

What kind of person made that commitment? I thought. He was as captivating to me as the ocean—vast and open, both beautiful and dangerous. We would end up dating and were doing just that for only a matter of weeks when a three-mile run in Barcelona called me home.

"You're doing what?" he had asked when I told him about my revelation. His mouth dropped open while we sat across from each other at the crew bar, sharing a bottle of wine, buzzed on both alcohol and intimacy.

THE DATE IS SET

"That's why I've been running so much lately." I told him, "I'm sore, but I feel stronger. Like I can just keep going!"

"You're serious? You're actually going to run across America?" He sat, amazed. "How?"

I shared my vision, and my words shaped an unlikely dream into something real—the thrill of a running tour across America with a purpose for my mother. "That would be amazing," he said. "You're so lucky. I've always wanted to tour the US."

"You should. Come with me," I offered impulsively. "We could tour the US together while I run!"

"Really? You think? That'd be crazy."

"It'd be great. The whole thing is crazy. Just think about it."

And he did. I left the ship, and he stayed. Months passed, and we continued considering my proposition during late-night phone calls halfway across the world from each other.

"You've never been to San Francisco, right?" I whispered into the phone in the dark.

"Yeah, never. I bet it's amazing."

"It is. The Wharf. Mission Street. There's so much there! And the Rocky Mountains are great too. I can't wait to run over them," I replied.

"The Statue of Liberty? I mean, babe, can you imagine how it will feel to see it after running all the way across the country?"

I could imagine it because I was. Each day while training, I'd run and think about what it'd be like. I'd eye motorhomes parked in driveways, parked at shopping centers, parked at the tire store up the street, and wonder which one I'd sleep in somewhere out west along a stretch of highway so desolate that the sky would twinkle with a thousand million stars.

And I told him these things too, painting how perfect it would be if he wanted to come as well—just an extension of our exotic relationship that had always resembled a vacation honeymoon. On ships, if we wanted to go skydiving together in Cancun, we did. Afterward, we'd eat tacos and drink beers, squishing warm sand between our toes before returning to work. The run wouldn't exactly be like this, but kind of.

"Think of all the places we'll see," we told each other. Just another adventure.

So, yes, there was a Nate. Of course, there was. There had always been a Nate for as far back as I'd been allowed to have one—Casey, Patrick, Peter, William, Nate—the line of notable boyfriends that captured my attention long enough to be a boyfriend. They were separated by a spattering of others in between—those ones being less notable. I was twenty-four and having fun, though not everyone approved. Namely, Steph, who eventually questioned my choices.

"Who? What happened to Tyler? I really liked him," she said to me while I recalled my latest fling.

"Well, you know," I replied.

As a serial monogamist, she wasn't interested in hearing it. "Forget it," she said. "I can't keep track. Just tell me when you're engaged."

Fine, I thought. *Let's talk when I'm thirty.*

After that, though, I couldn't help but feel a bit careless. Was something wrong with me that caused me to discard perfectly good relationships? Why was I uninterested so quickly? Maybe love, I wondered, was about accepting annoyances like the irritating way one drank through a straw and choosing to stay anyway. Soon after Steph's criticism, I met Nate in a bar, just like my parents had done. Dreaming up these things with him, lying in his arms on a deck chair on the fourteenth floor of a cruise ship, felt magical, destined.

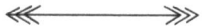

"WE MADE IT, BABE," Nate said to me now, turning off the engine of the motorhome, sitting at my side in the driving cab. "We're here."

Here was the home of Greg and Michelle Turner in Oakdale, California. A man from Milwaukee read about me in the newspaper and knew someone who lived near my start. He emailed me to ask if I would be interested in staying with them when I arrived, and now here we were.

Nate parked the motorhome precariously in front of the Turners' house on the kind of slope that the Bay Area was known for, with

THE DATE IS SET

the wheels turned in toward the curb—rather crash the beast into a house than careen it down the hill into traffic if the brakes failed.

The beast was a 1994 Ford Class A motorhome, thirty feet in length. The inside was drenched in a powder-blue hue—blue canvas curtains, blue velour couch, blue worn carpet that covered every inch of the floor. She came to me six short weeks prior when my aunt hosted a polka pancake breakfast as a fundraiser in middle-of-nowhere Wisconsin.

"A family at the event knows someone with a motorhome, honey," she said through the phone. It sounded like an unlikely source, but then I found myself headed there in February with my father to pick it up. I drove it home, bouncing down the highway with the winter winds beating its broadsides, insisting to my father that I do it myself because I needed to know how. My hands white-knuckled the steering wheel the entire three-hour drive until I arrived home and told Nate that driving it to California would be no problem at all, which didn't exactly end up being true.

"Okay, what do we need?" I said, standing up from the passenger seat directly into the living space. The driving area sat atop the engine in front of a full-picture window, like a bus. A thirteen-inch box TV with a VCR player was embedded into the dash. The vehicle was vintage and full of promise. That—plus everything we stuffed in her before we left Wisconsin: eleven pairs of identical running shoes, sweat-wicking shorts, running skirts, tops, tanks, socks, a massive box of bulk medical supplies—gauze, break-and-use ice packs, athletic tape, and Band-Aids; unopened supplements—powders and pills wrapped in their boxes that I had yet to try, my hydration belt with its neon green water bottles, running visors and hats, winter caps, running gloves, one pair of Gore-Tex water-resistant running shoes, base layers and a winter running jacket, fleece lined running pants, and wool socks, a fuchsia pink fitness watch with its companion heart rate monitor, headphones and an iPod mini, two pairs of jeans, casual T-shirts, a pair of sweatpants, two hoodies and one pair of black dress pants with a polyester silk top (for dinners and special events), a laundry basket filled with new blankets, towels, washcloths, bed linens, shampoo and bathing items (all with their tags still on), two small inch plants, a MacBook laptop, my BlackBerry smartphone, a library of books—*The Secret*, *The Traveler's Gift*, *The Slight Edge*, *Eat Pray Love*, and a poster of Jackie Joyner-Kersee looking lean and badass clearing a track hurdle with the words *Run Like A Girl* printed above her.

I looked at the boxes and bags of these things crammed into all the spaces—under the couch, behind the swivel chair, under the dinette table, and atop its bench seats—and the clutter made me uneasy. For me, everything had to have a place, and nothing was just so. We had left Wisconsin for the coast in haste, throwing these supplies into open spaces because there was no time left and a plethora of other things to do. This would be our home for the next 190 days, and I felt an itchy pull to stay within the vehicle and begin organizing immediately. But for now, I'd have to leave it. We were at the Turners', ready to meet them for the first time and sleep in their spare bedroom for the next two days. On the third morning here, I'd start my run across America.

"Let's go say hi," Nate suggested. "I need to stretch my legs. We can come back later for anything we need."

Stepping onto their front lawn through the only door to the vehicle, a hinged opening on the passenger side, I glanced back at her exterior. It *was* a dull white color with faded blue swooshes bleached by the sun, but we had that covered with a vinyl wrap before we left. The words "Ashley's 3,200 Mile Run Across America For Multiple Sclerosis" stretched across the top in giant orange letters. It was a bold statement—a commitment of unimaginable miles—but it didn't shake me. I had endured the misery of training through endless stretches of road for hours at a time, and I was here all the same. By now, I knew how it might feel to do this. My first marathon nearly brought me to my knees.

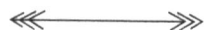

"**YOU'RE RUNNING A MARATHON?** When?" asked my father.

"Now," I said. I had poked my head through the doorframe of his office and announced I was running a marathon. I'd just

THE DATE IS SET

completed another chapter in the *Ultramarathon Man* book I was reading and, feeling inspired, decided that now was the time I would finally run twenty-six miles.

I had been home for four weeks already since leaving the cruise ship. It was a touch after 10:00 a.m. on a vibrant March day, and spring's fresh energy pulled me to the road. Winter receded to bursts of warmth flirting through the air, challenging me to test the ideas I absorbed at night reading alone in the dark, my bedside lamp aglow upon words written by ultramarathon runners, a crazed type of people I had never heard of who ran distances north of a marathon—50k, 50 miles, 100 miles, 136 miles through Death Valley in July. My pulse quickened at their stories. I saw myself within the pages.

"Where are you going? What are you taking with you?" my father asked.

"I'm running to Pewaukee Lake, around it, and back. I mapped it out. It's seven miles to the lake and twelve miles around. I don't need anything. Just my shoes," I told him with a smile.

Dean Karnazes, the author of the book, hadn't taken supplies on his first thirty-mile run. He left a bar after dark and ran in his dirty garden shoes. Certainly, I was more qualified than that.

"I'll be back in, like, four hours," I said. Then I turned to go, making no fuss about running a marathon for the first time.

I didn't need food, a water bottle, money, or even my phone. It was running, just running! Of course, I would run a marathon now. It would be no problem. If I wanted to run across America, I would need to do this. Not once, but many times over. I read no blogs. I called no runners. Instead, I tied on my shoes and left the house.

Mile after easy mile, I ran from my parents' place, down Lookout Hill, then northwest toward the lake. My stride was light and steady. My arms eased in motion.

Look at this, I thought, *I'm running a marathon. How lovely. How plain.*

An hour later, still moving at a comfortable pace, my parents drove by and honked the car horn. "Way to go, Ashbee!" my father shouted. It was an unexpected surprise. They came to watch. I waved at my very own cheer station, then leapfrogged them every few miles—Mom clapping enthusiastically from the open car window and Dad on the horn each time I passed.

Nate would do the same, I imagined, giving support just like this. He'd crew me on my run across the country. He'd lace up his shoes and run at my side. He'd say things like, "Way to go, babe!" and give me a kiss. I smiled at the thought.

The miles ticked by—seven, then nine, then thirteen. Halfway. A distance I had run twice before.

Soon after, my route took me off the streets and onto a tree-lined recreation path. I gave my parents a wave and then ran along through miles fourteen, fifteen, sixteen, and seventeen until the trail merged onto the street again. I expected to see my parents with a honk and a wave. Yet, the road was barren.

I slowed to a walk and looked around at the empty street. *They must be just over that hill*, I thought, running again. When I crested the hill, the street was empty. I slowed to a walk. *Where are they?*

I turned to look behind me. Nothing. Then, up ahead, searching in both directions like a spinning top. Nothing.

I was hopeful for their encouragement, but truthfully, my mouth had dried to the consistency of sandpaper. I had been running for two hours and thirty-seven minutes, according to my watch, and I needed a drink—water, Gatorade, something, anything.

I put my hands on my knees and hung my head. My stomach let out an audible growl.

I wasn't thirsty, and I wasn't hungry. These words are too comfortable to describe what I was feeling, like verbs I'd use to recall what might prompt me to move from the couch to the kitchen. This was not that. This was a sudden, ruthless emptiness. I felt fine until I didn't, becoming ravaged in an instant.

I'd eat a whole bushel of bananas, a double-stacked quarter-pound burger with pickles, a chocolate milkshake, a bag of salt-and-vinegar chips, a box of Oreos. I'd stick my face under a fast-food soda fountain and not care who saw.

But I was nowhere near these things. In fact, I was eight miles

away from any of it, which was at least another hour and a half of running. Likely more.
Alone.
Just running.
How lovely. How plain.
How fucked. *Goddamnit.*
My eyes stared between my aching feet at the concrete, thick and heavy like my legs, while considering that my parents may have actually gone home. Maybe they got hungry. Maybe Mom needed to use the bathroom. The last time they saw me, like all the times before it, I was strong. I waved at them with a smile, then ambled gleefully down the recreation trail like a leprechaun skipping down a rainbow. Dean ran thirty miles out the door of a bar in garden tennis shoes without training? How? Did I remember the story correctly? Damn it, Dean. What the fuck?
Fuck Dean. Fuck this.
"Fuuuuuck!" I groaned aloud, finally admitting to myself that the fastest way out was to continue. To end it, I'd have to endure it.
Running again in a weakened shuffle, my shoes scrubbed the cement of its dirt like a street sweeper brushing the ground. My shoulders withered. My body folded. I ran until I couldn't, then I walked until I could run. A slow, deep ache crawled up my calves and inched its way to my hamstrings and lower back. It was the burn of depleting muscle—fibers tearing, tissue dissolving. Hours of running without fuel and my body was breaking down what it could for energy. I felt the unbearable anguish of myself literally consuming me.
Okay. What doesn't hurt? I asked myself. Taking inventory, not much. My arms ached, and my legs screamed. My skin rubbed itself raw. *Concentrate on the motion,* I told myself. So I did.
I heard the impact of my feet against the pavement. One foot. Then the other.
I felt the balanced swinging of my arms. One forward. The other back.
I sensed the air move through my lungs. Breathe in, expanding. Breathe out, release.

Rhythmic and soothing. A lullaby on repeat.

No doubt, I felt famished and lonely and saturated in pain, more so than I ever had before. But the melody of the motion centered me. *How many times has Mom experienced something like this? Is this what her MS symptoms feel like?* I caught glimpses of her cringe silently on bad days, clutching the couch and squeezing her eyes shut when she didn't know I was looking. She never made a thing of her symptoms. Rather, she went on and rarely complained. The thought of it propelled me forward. My suffering was self-inflicted. Hers was undeserving.

I went on for miles, dragging myself along—controlling my thoughts, reframing my pain within the context of my mother's—when a mirage appeared. It was a forest green sedan on the road ahead. I squinted. *Was it moving?* Yes, it was getting bigger. My knees buckled in recognition. It was them—my parents!

"Daaaaaad! Dad. I'm hurting. Bad. Can you get me Gatorade? Food?" I blurted out when they finally pulled to my side.

Minutes later, I smashed two bananas in my face, then every drop of a cold blue Gatorade. A tidal wave of silk washed over me, from my head all the way to my feet. It was sugar coursing through my veins.

"Ahhhhhhhhhh!" I exhaled. My cells pulsed in both misery and relief, raw and alive. To recover, I took the weight off my feet by lying my head and chest across the car's trunk.

"Honey, you should get in," my mom said from the open car window. "You've done enough for today."

I stared at the road ahead and considered getting in with just three miles left—to lie down in the back across the plush fabric, resting my body and feeling accomplished about running twenty-three miles. But what would that mean for me now on this path toward my goal of running across America? To give in so close to the finish?

I lifted my head and, with it, peeled my body off the car like a used Band-Aid—dirty, limp, and worn.

"Thanks, Mom," I said. "But I'll keep going. I'm training to run to New York, not New Jersey."

And at that, I ran home.

THE DATE IS SET

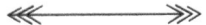

"**WE BOUGHT IT ON** a whim," Michelle said of their multimillion-dollar, five-bedroom home after they welcomed us inside and helped us get our things settled in the guest room. "We were strolling through the neighborhood on a Sunday, peeking through open houses, and knew we had to have it."

I nodded, staring at the panoramic view that overlooked a stretch of bay water from their top floor, and wondered what that would be like—to walk into a home unencumbered and buy it because I could. I felt a pang of envy. They had everything I thought I wanted.

"Here, we have one more thing to show you," Greg said, moving toward the stairs.

On the main level in the kitchen, I looked out another window at a much less impressive sight—a used white Toyota Camry parked in the back alleyway. "Our kids learned how to drive with this car. It's a little dinged up, but it's in good shape."

I peered at it, mildly interested. What an odd transition.

"It's been sitting for a year. We keep meaning to donate it to charity but haven't made time. You're a 501(c)3 nonprofit, correct?"

Chills ran up my back. I was—a byproduct of me contacting MS organizations for partnership, but only receiving general do-it-yourself fundraising pages instead. My event wasn't a simple DIY. It was a whole thing. I was going to raise $500,000, and I wanted every dollar that was donated to fund my mission to support research for a cure. Acquiring sponsorship to fund the event—the fuel, the food, and other expenses—was a major facet of my plan from the start. As a twenty-four-year-old with little savings, I couldn't pay for the cost myself. I needed help, and I needed money. One year prior, while at home training for the endeavor, I told my parents just that.

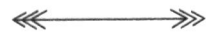

"**I THINK I HAVE** to start a charity," I said, plopping down heavily on the couch next to my mom and letting out a sigh.

Dad was in the recliner. *The Price Is Right* wheel was dinging on the TV.

"Why's that?" he asked, taking his eyes from the screen to look at me.

"The MS organizations I've contacted aren't able to commit to the partnership I need for sponsorships. I need tax exemption. They're sending me general fundraising pages."

"So, what's it take to start one?"

"That's the problem," I said. "The application is $700, the document is more than twenty-eight pages long, and the internet says to get a lawyer to fill it out, which costs like $10,000. It's way too much."

Thumbing through the paperwork with my parents, we decided I could complete it myself. "It's kind of like a business plan," my dad pointed out. "If you get through all this work, we'll cover the fee as our first donation to your nonprofit."

I smiled, relieved. Until I started the work.

Weeks passed.

I trudged my way through, page after page, picking them up and setting them down so much that the edges wore thin and ink got smudged. I cross-checked the instructions dozens of times and created the framework that would become the charity.

What was the organization's mission, history, intended budget, and giving profile? I made it all up (the budget being so far off that it made me sweat the first time I filled the motorhome with gas).

Who was the board? Three people were required. I wrote down my dad, myself, and a friend.

How would the funds be distributed, and where was the main office? I penned another charity as recipient and then looked around my childhood bedroom. Does this qualify as a main office? I wrote my parents' home address.

When I was finally done, I clipped a $700 check scribbled in my father's handwriting to its pages, stuffed it in a cinched pack, and carried it on my back while I ran the 4.3 miles from my parents'

THE DATE IS SET

home to the post office for training. I dropped my budding dreams into the depths of a dark metal box, shutting the trap door closed with a *clang*, and ran home.

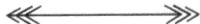

SITTING IN THE TURNERS' Toyota, which was now my charity's Toyota, I rubbed my hands across the top of the smooth leather steering wheel. They knew we needed a support vehicle because I had asked them where we could buy an inexpensive moped, which was my cheap solution to getting to and from the route each day from the camper. In the Camry now, I realized how silly that plan was. Me, loading up my running gear, food, and supplies into a moped basket. Nate, driving down the highway with me teetering on the back, to and from the route every day after running a full marathon, through rain, snow, and all the weather we would experience until we reached New York. Really? I chuckled at myself, shaking my head.

Even in my lumbering, I felt conviction. Here I was, with a family I was introduced to by a man I had never met, sitting in a car they intended for a charity the whole year I trained, and then I showed up, having created a charity that needed a vehicle. How else could one explain these remarkable coincidences except to believe that it was all meant to be? It was oddly reminiscent of the RV parked out front, which appeared to me just a mere forty-six days before I was scheduled to leave for the start of the run.

"We don't have a motorhome," Nate had argued. "We're supposed to leave next month. We need to discuss pushing the date back."

I would not. I held the line. "If we change the date now, that means we never believed it was there for us in the first place. You know what I'm talking about," I said. "You gave me the book."

The book was called *The Secret*, and it was a favorite of his, which he handed to me shortly after we started dating. It contextualized what I had already learned from my parents—that intention was a tangible force. Like when my mother's abilities fluctuated from fluid, to manageable, to crippling and back again. The good days would string together one after another until they were abruptly swallowed by immobility. During an episode, she would lie on the couch for days at a time in between trips to the bathroom. My parents bought no wheelchair for help, installed no guardrails for balance.

Without equipment, my father would wrestle the deadweight of her body onto a cobalt blue office chair with wheels. She'd wobble around, ever-present yet as cooperative as a hundred-pound bag of pudding, and he'd push her to the bathroom. Then he'd hoist her to the toilet, let her do her business, then hoist her back to the chair and onto the couch again. Again and again until her function returned. This bathroom routine happened often during a relapse on account of the disease's effects on her nervous system—her having little control over sensations, resulting in an accident if she waited too long. During the daytime, she wore underwear to preserve her dignity. At night, she conceded to adult diapers on account of all the laundry.

From the outside, this office chair routine would look like madness. Why not just get a wheelchair?

"Ashley," my father explained, "what you allow continues. If we put her in a wheelchair, we may just never get her out."

It was a lot of work. A *lot* of work. But it was a clearing for mobility to return, and they'd hold space for it as long as they could manage. MS could be cruelly unpredictable—its debilitating symptoms sometimes receding, sometimes not, and never knowing which it would be. Still, their intention remained.

And now I had myself a guy who believed in this way of thinking too.

"This day holds just as much promise as the ones before it. You know this, Nate," I encouraged him. "It'll happen."

"I know," he agreed. "It's just we're running out of time. We don't have a motorhome. It makes me anxious. What are we going to do?"

"We can't think about what we don't have. We have to focus on what we know," I said, grabbing his shoulders. "We proceed, expecting it to appear. Okay?"

THE DATE IS SET

He nodded his head yes. "Okay."

"The date is set. March 16, we leave Wisconsin. March 22, I run across the Golden Gate Bridge. Right?"

He stood tall. "Right."

And that's exactly what happened.

CHAPTER FIVE

Gateway

ON MARCH 22, 2010, I stood at a crack in the asphalt. "This looks good to me," I said of my starting line in a parking lot at the foot of the Golden Gate Bridge.

It was an odd day and time to start an endurance run by all endurance event standards—noon on a Monday. When I picked the date a year earlier, beginning at the top of the week felt right to me, not considering that people would want to be there. I pushed my early morning start time back to midday to encompass a lunchtime running group—the four runners with me now—and to accommodate a crowd that would look good for the news, which was there as well.

"If you could run around this building here, I'll be over there," the cameraman from Channel 4 had instructed me an hour earlier, "and then I can get a great shot of you starting past the bridge and running up those steps over there."

I nodded, retaining his words like high school geometry. Moments before, I had parked the RV horizontally across four parking spaces and cut the engine. People had already started gathering. While talking with the cameraman, their presence pulled at my attention. He gave instructions. I waved hello to my aunt.

The start of my run was very much me, deep and unfussed. Beginning a run across America at an iconic landmark by lining up at a fault in the pavement was exactly that. People were drawn to the motorhome because that was the only thing that marked my presence—a thirty-foot vehicle with my nonprofit's logo four feet tall and five feet wide across both sides.

"It has to be something gender-neutral." I had said of the logo to my friend a year prior, after she'd handed me a few sketches of a female running. "It can't be about a girl running. It has to be about anyone running for MS."

I still had no idea what the charity had to offer others, but I felt a pull to build something for any runner. So when people arrived at the Crissy Field parking area to a lot filled with cars, they went to the motorhome stretched across four spaces that was decorated with a cause logo—a road fading into the letters *M* and *S* with the words "Run The US" below it.

"Ten... nine... eight... seven... six..." Nate called out, leading the crowd in a countdown chant. "Five... four... three... two... one... go!"

I clicked start on my watch and took off, running down the length of the parking lot that led to a paved, narrow path. It would wind us up through dense brush past a scenic overlook, then onto a pedestrian pathway that stretched the length of the Golden Gate Bridge. I felt anxious and light, thrilled to finally be running across America.

Seven days prior, Nate and I had left Wisconsin and driven four days straight to the coast. The spaces in between driving were used to read the vehicle's manual to learn how to use it, and my legs hadn't seen a decent run in over a week. The feeling of striding now had me elated. My arms loosened into ease. My legs cycled in motion.

I was doing it!

I was running across America on the exact day I marked boldly on a calendar twelve months prior.

Except, now, what I heard was... stop?

"Stop! Stop! Come back!" the cameraman from the news yelled.

I halted and looked at my back to see him awkwardly running at me, his bulky camera jostling back and forth atop his shoulder like a vintage boom box.

"You were supposed to run around that building," he said,

arriving at me a couple hundred yards from my start, out of breath and pointing to the place he had shown me an hour earlier.

"Oh, sorry," I said, chuckling, feeling my cheeks flush with embarrassment. "I forgot."

"Can you come back and start again?"

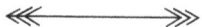

IT HAD BEEN AN unhurried morning—having breakfast, organizing our things, Nate documenting the notable day by coming into the bathroom unannounced while I rinsed toothpaste from the sink.

"Okay, so, it's the morning of Ashley's big run across America. I've just woken up to see how she's feeling, what kind of emotions are running through her head, and the expectations for the day," he said, pointing a Nikon camera at my face.

"I'm feeling wonderful, uh. Just another day in San Francisco." I told the lens, saying the first thing that came to my mind, feeling uninteresting and silly, used toothpaste froth on my hands.

I had gotten up and brushed my teeth in a steady calm, yielding my energy for the place it mattered most. I controlled my thoughts, halting them from hyping the day into something astronomical that I could not achieve, like literally thinking about running 3,200 miles over the next six months. I wasn't thinking about my "big run across America" because I wasn't doing that today. Today, I was running seventeen miles in San Francisco. I had no profound emotions about doing that because it was an obtainable distance that I would simply do in an iconic setting. I uneventfully cleaned my teeth—prepared for the long game—when Nate came in and asked me how I felt about eating the moon.

He shut the camera down and looked at me, expecting more.

I mirrored his gaze and walked past him toward my bag. People could expect what they wanted. The miles owned me now. Except that wasn't fully true, with me running back and forth in the parking lot for forty minutes while the cameraman produced shots for the news—around the building, past the building, up the stairs, stop here and wait, now again but like this.

GATEWAY

"Sorry." I blushed at the runners at my side. I had told them that we'd cover at least three miles before they had to return to work, and now they were wasting their afternoon run doing circles with me in a parking lot.

I could see Nate just yards from where I stood, my aunt and uncle, a childhood friend, a group from the local MS organization, all milling about near the motorhome. I was grateful for the media and had gotten used to it over the year I'd promoted the endeavor, but doing this now, so close to the bridge after envisioning it for more than a year, made me feel like a thoroughbred clamoring in a starting gate. *Just let me fucking go.*

The weather was perfect—a pleasant sixty-degree day with clear skies and the occasional dollop of cloud floating by. I wanted to jump up and grab one, put it in my pocket to remember the day by. But I hadn't wanted to collect items at the start or finish, something I explained to the runners now.

"Did you gather a bit of sand and water? Something from here that you'll get again when you finish?" a woman in the group had asked.

The cameraman adjusted his lens for the next shot.

"Actually, it's the bridges I'm drawn to," I told her, looking at it—a massive orange suspension bridge that felt more like a gateway than a beginning. I likened the platform of steel to the same as I had always used running—a solid structure providing safe passage over what lurked below.

Opened to the public in 1937, the Golden Gate Bridge was almost two miles in length and connected the city of San Francisco to Marin County, where I was headed. I hadn't thought to look at its direction when I picked it as my start. Just that it was a famous point on the coast that fit my route. But looking at a map more closely weeks ago, I realized I couldn't actually run east right away—the bridge was built north to south. To use it as my starting point, I'd have to run north around San Pablo Bay first, through Marin County, and into Napa. Once there, fifty miles or so later, then I could head east. It didn't bother me.

I've always wanted to see Napa! I told myself.

"Okay." The cameraman waved, checking his footage one last time. "I got it. It'll air tonight. Good luck."

"Finally," I exhaled to the group.

We ascended the winding path and took off along the pedestrian walkway. The towering uprights soared into the sky. A thrill fluttered in my stomach.

"So, how did you pick the route?" a marathoner to my right asked.

"I mostly picked places I wanted to see," I replied, striding at a comfortable pace. "I lived in Denver for a while, so that made the list. And then I wanted to get as close to home as possible, so that's why I picked Chicago. With those two cities as anchors, that really pulled the route north."

"But what about the actual roads?" he replied. "Like, the ones you'll go on today? It must have taken forever to map it out."

"Not really. I use my BlackBerry," I answered. "I pull up Google Maps, plug in the points, and run." The phone was clipped to my shorts in a lavender-colored case that shimmered in the sunlight.

"Are you serious? Like, you haven't studied the roads?" he asked.

"No, not really. That kind of took a back seat to finding a motorhome and getting a sponsor. They're roads, I'll figure them out," I replied.

I was aware how I came across—naive, overly optimistic, a "Pollyanna," one reporter described me. I read one book about someone else's run across America—David McGillivray's 1978 run, the current race director of the prestigious Boston Marathon. Before his crossing, admittedly being a precise and calculated person, he spent four years mapping each and every road. Admirable, but that was *not* me.

I also spoke to one other person who had done it as well—a man who reached out to me, insisting on a phone call. He talked for nearly an hour about how difficult it would be for me to find a sponsor to pay for everything and that I should expect my run to go mostly unnoticed because, as he found out during his run, people weren't interested in such a long event, so, he just wanted me to know.

"I wouldn't sponsor him either," I told my dad afterward. "What a grump."

My run would be my own, I decided. Everyone else could keep their baggage, something I tried to explain to the runners now, raising my voice so the group could hear me over the six-lane highway that paralleled the sidewalk to our left. A suspension cable, the width of a sequoia, sloped upward before us.

"Yeah, I'm not really worried about getting injured," I replied to another question. "I've never had a running injury before, so I'm not going to bring one on by thinking about it now."

"But you've also never run this many miles before."

"I'm not breaking any records," I offered. "I'll do the entire crossing like this at a talking pace."

A woman in a light-blue top looked at her GPS watch. "We're at about nine-twenties," she said, stating our pace per mile in minutes and seconds. "You're going to hold this the whole way?"

"I won't know. I didn't get a GPS watch," I said. "I'm wearing a heart rate monitor to track calories and time. Some days, I'll run faster if I feel like it. Other days, I'll run slower. I'll walk when I need to and just enjoy the road."

"I couldn't do it," admitted another. "I've done three marathons, and each time, I'm wrecked for days after."

"Yeah, but ultrarunning is different," I offered. "Running twenty-six miles nonstop as fast as you can is hard on your body. I'm not doing that. I'll run about fifteen miles or so every morning, taking breaks at the car every hour to eat and rehydrate. Then I'll rest for lunch, eat, maybe take a nap, and go back out for another hour or two in the afternoon." I squeezed a squirt of fruit punch sports drink into my mouth from my handheld water bottle. "The pace and nutrition and rest are what make it doable."

"Yeah." The man thought for a moment. "I still couldn't do it." The group, including me, laughed.

"So what do you eat when you run?" another runner asked.

"Everything," I said, getting a few chuckles of my own. "Bananas, peanut-butter-and-jelly sandwiches, pickles, trail mix. I love salt-and-vinegar chips. Basically, whatever I'm craving. My body knows what it needs. It'll tell me. I actually gained weight on purpose while training to have extra fat for the crossing. I'm eight pounds heavier than normal right now."

"How'd you manage that with all the running?"

"It's actually easier than you'd think with ultrarunning. For me, it was about finding a pace that I could maintain for a really long period of time. Your body acclimates and gets really efficient. Adding weight then was about adding calories after doing a run that my body is really efficient at. I'd do five to eight miles every day, longer runs on the weekends, a handful of ultras, cross-training. This, right now, is actually my final phase of training. I'll keep the miles lower for the first third of the crossing, around twenty each day, until I get over the Rocky Mountains. Once I hit the Midwest, then I'll run closer to thirty, maybe more. By that time, my body'll be able to handle it."

I outlined my plan, as I had done countless times before, and took in the moment, finally making my way across the bridge. Groups of tourists strolled along the path, taking pictures of Alcatraz Island in the distance. A gentle breeze blew across my skin. A tiny white triangle bobbed upon the water below, heading out to sea. A seagull gliding along its canvas sail.

"And Chris told me you ran your first marathon just a couple months ago? Is that true?" Eric asked. He was the brother of a race director I knew in Milwaukee and the only runner from this group who would stay with me for the next ten miles.

"Well, I mean, technically, yes." I laughed. "I ran the distance plenty of times during training, but for racing, I skipped the marathon and did fifty milers instead. Chris's indoor marathon in January was my first 'race' marathon."

"You didn't race a marathon before you raced a fifty miler?" the woman in blue asked.

I shrugged and nodded my head.

"Why not?"

"I dunno," I answered. "I just didn't feel the need to."

"And what's an indoor marathon?" she asked.

"It's ninety-four laps around a couple hockey rinks at the Petit National Ice Center in Milwaukee," Eric explained. "My brother founded the race as a way to host a marathon in Wisconsin in January."

"You ran your first marathon race on a *track*?" the guy asked.

I shrugged. "I did everything hard and boring I could think of to prepare for this. If the weather sucked, I was outside running. If it was crazy hot or freezing cold or gale-force winds, I went running for as long as I could. So when Chris asked if I wanted to run a marathon and also a half marathon on a track back-to-back in the same weekend, I was all for it. Plus, my parents got to sit in the stands and watch me the whole time. It was actually pretty fun."

"Oh! I bet they loved that," the other woman added. "How is your mom?"

I sighed inaudibly. It was the question I grew to hate.

I knew people meant well, but I wondered if they wanted the truth—that things were difficult, that she lived with significant disability, my father was her main caregiver, and there was a lot of stress on him and their finances. That, at any moment, they could lose everything if her health plummeted. Often, I overheard my father on the phone, working on insurance coverage for her, again, after the forms were filed, but someone didn't allocate them correctly, again, trying to get her monthly $6,000 medication cost covered.

My parents' net worth was healthy on paper, but their monthly income staggered under the weight of a family-run business, supporting the astronomical cost of her health care. It wasn't just the MS medication. It was all the others used to manage her symptoms as well. She took eleven pills each day, plus a shot, and most of them came with adverse side effects. She had four root canals in one year before my dad realized it was a new medicine causing the decay. I'm sure there was help somewhere, but who knew how to find it? Hundreds of thousands of people were living with the disease, with limited resources to help. My effort to raise half a million dollars was a drop in the bucket, and I knew it. Having MS was not easy or inexpensive, and for some people, it was unmanageable. My parents were actually lucky, if one would call it that, all things considered.

I said none of this. It invoked a look of sadness followed by an awkward silence that no one knew how to fill, including me. Instead, I kept running and gave my father's token response: "She's doing okay. She has her good days and her bad days, but we're making it work."

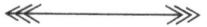

INTO MARIN COUNTY, THE route took Eric and me through the quaint town of Sausalito, a cute waterside village that reminded me much of Nice, a port city in France. We had crossed the bridge, reaching the point where the other runners had to return. Eric and I waved them goodbye and continued on.

Weaving up and down the hills along the shore, I looked out upon the teetering sailboats clustered near the piers and wondered who owned them—their empty white masts looking like hors d'oeuvre toothpicks wobbling on the water. Someone anchored their boat, then made their way to a restaurant patio along the water to join others sipping mimosas in the sunlight. For a moment, I wished to be them—wealthy and buzzed, drinking in bubbles and sunshine on a Monday afternoon.

"So, where'd you get the motorhome?" Eric asked, bringing me back to the run. We departed the Sausalito sidewalk and merged onto a paved recreation path along the water.

"Ha, that's a good story. It all came about thanks to maple syrup."

"What?" Eric laughed, giving me a funny look.

"We got it donated by a family about six weeks ago at a fundraiser my aunt put together, a polka pancake breakfast at a Lions Club in Wildrose, Wisconsin."

"Yeesh. Six weeks. That's cutting it close," he replied. "What were you going to do if that didn't happen?"

"Push a stroller," I said, laughing. "But, you know, thanks to Joe and Mary Ann, I don't have to."

"Why do I get the feeling that you've never used a motorhome before this?" he poked lightly.

I just smiled. "I learn by doing."

The recreation path was beautiful—vibrant marshes of reeds swaying in the seaside valley of rolling hills—marine air filling my senses with salty freshness—a furry ocean mammal flipping along the surface. It came to me then that I was covering miles I wouldn't ever see again on this journey, and the thought of it made me feel light and bold. These subtleties kept me present, searing a feeling of adventure into the moment.

"Nate should be just up ahead," I said, pointing to an area that intersected with the path, 7.7 miles from where we began. "I am ready to eat."

The spot had been decided upon earlier that morning while Nate and I reviewed the route quickly in the parking lot at the bridge. We dropped a pin on his map, and then I walked to my starting line, forgetting to grab snacks to carry along. After running around for the reporter before crossing the bridge, it was after 2:00 p.m. now, and my stomach growled. I hadn't eaten since breakfast.

Instead of seeing Nate and the motorhome filled with the salt-and-vinegar chips that I had been craving, a woman I had just met opened the Camry's driver's side door.

"Hi, I brought refreshments," Kristina said, holding up a convenience store bag. "Nate's kind of stuck and couldn't get here just yet."

"Stuck? What do you mean?" I asked.

"Well, he took a wrong turn with the RV and went down a one-way in the city. He asked me to come meet you. When I left, he and your uncle were still trying to figure out how to turn around."

I looked back toward San Francisco as if I could see it with my own eyes. He was still back in the city?

"Does he need me?" I offered. I couldn't help but want to fix it.

"No, no. I think he and your uncle have it figured out. Your aunt was directing traffic while Nate reversed down the street. He felt pretty good about meeting you at your finish today."

Pretty good? What did that mean? There were seven miles remaining between me and my finish at a park in San Rafael. I thought it would be easy to find. Now, I wasn't so sure.

"Here." She smiled, handing over the plastic bag, "I picked these up on the way here." In it was a variety of granola bars and a cherry Gatorade.

"Thanks," I said, hoping to hide my disappointment. My tummy rumbled, thinking of the plethora of chips in the motorhome.

They were the perfect amount of crunchiness and flavor. I devoured the kettle kind, the ones that were a bit thicker and crispier. I'd pull apart the sealed top and smell a waft of greasy potato crisps. Putting one into my mouth, I'd savor the seasoning of salt with a rush of saliva. Being on the verge of parched, this would be delightful. Then I'd hear the crunch, a lively sound, while my tongue moved around the freshness of vinegar. I'd swallow, then reach my hand into the bag for more, eating until my mouth felt raw.

Instead, I pushed a dry strawberry Quaker bar between my lips and tried to feel satisfied.

In all honesty, I was exhausted and looking for the chips to bring me life. The activity of the day had taken its toll—the late start, meeting groups of people, embracing those I knew, being introduced to those I didn't, sharing my story, preparing to run. Each exchange took effort, and the lack of nutrition on my part made it worse. Miles that should have felt easy didn't. My hips throbbed. My backside ached. I needed to eat a heap of calories, ice my knees, and lie on my back for a bit. But first, I had to run seven more miles.

Get to the park, I told myself after Kristina and then Eric peeled away. *Nate will be there waiting for you. You can have chips and ice for your knees then.* I imagined him standing in anticipation at the edge of the park, searching for me. He was worried, of course, after having gotten stuck and not being at the stop to meet me. He'd clap and holler, as my parents would have, cheering me on to the end of my first day.

I imagined this scene and ran. The bay continued to sparkle in the sunlight. Seagulls cackled in flight. There was plenty to enjoy while I moved along, leaving the disappointment behind.

That is, until I got there.

Arriving at the park on the edge of a business district, I came upon our meeting place completely unnoticed. The sidewalk lined a baseball field, where, across the open grass, the motorhome sat on the other side of the park, the length of a football field away, which, in that moment, felt quite far.

My hunger was at an anxious level. My throat felt raw from all the talking, and my insides roared. Between me and the vehicles, Nate kicked a soccer ball back and forth with my uncle.

Finally, "Hey! Babe!" he shouted, kicking the ball one last time and coming my way. "What a crazy day. Did Kristina tell you? I took a wrong turn down a one-way and had to stop. The RV was way too big. People were honking. It was so stressful."

"I heard," I said, continuing my way toward the RV, trying to control myself, exhausted and famished. Stuck? Stressed about driving? I had just run seventeen miles with twenty more to run tomorrow and the thousands that remained thereafter. Was he concerned with taking care of me or not?

Surely, there's food ready for you inside, I told myself. It would be a buffet organized on the table, just as they did at ultramarathon races. A peanut-butter-and-jelly sandwich next to a mound of salt-and-vinegar chips. A chocolate chip cookie, maybe two. Bananas. Chilled grapes. Chocolate milk.

Coming into an aid station at a race, the volunteers would cheer for you over AC/DC's "Thunderstruck" playing on their portable speakers, smiling and asking if you wanted chicken noodle soup (that they had prepared at the perfect drinkable temperature) or if you'd rather have some pretzels? Here, we have three different drinks for you: soda down there, electrolytes in the middle, and water over here. And, also, give me your water bottle. I'll fill it for you. You look great, really great! Keep it up!

You could look like absolute shit, dragging your ass to the table, dirty and sore, and they'd still say it all the same. Running for hours on end wasn't easy—all that time inside your head with the least of physical, emotional, or environmental imbalances tipping you toward quitting, and they knew it. They'd see you through as best they could, filling your barren cup with their cheer and pushing you down the trail. Sometimes you needed it; sometimes you didn't. Either way, it was always there.

I pulled the motorhome door open and stepped inside.

The table was empty.

CHAPTER SIX

Tracks

THE NEXT MORNING, I awoke in the motorhome to Nate beside me in bed and a man sleeping on the futon couch ten feet from us in the living quarters.

I gently pulled my covers back and crept toward the kitchen, letting Nate wake slowly. Sitting down at the bench seat farthest from the futon, me in my sweats, the man in his canvas cargo pants and yesterday's shirt, I asked him about his night.

"Hey, how'd you sleep?" I said quietly.

"Good," he said, rubbing his face, voice groggy. "I've certainly slept in worse spots."

"Good," I beamed, wanting him to feel comfortable.

It was 8:00 a.m. already, quite late to be waking to run twenty miles, but day one had been hectic. The night before, both the man and Nate had convinced me that it'd be best to ease into the morning. "Well, I'll make some tea, and then we can talk about the route. Did you get any decent shots yesterday?"

His name was Spade, and he was the event's photographer. We met just four weeks prior, and for the next six months, he'd be sleeping on the couch.

Like the leaves falling off the trees, the months had fallen off the calendar—I had arrived home from the ship in February, then came March when I ran my first marathon, April into May, when I ran my first ultramarathon, then June into July, when I received a letter from the IRS incorporating my nonprofit, August, September, October, into November, when I rushed into Nate's arms at Milwaukee International Airport, December into January, when our motorhome appeared, until finally it was February again, one month until my start date, and the money to pay for it came too.

"Can I speak to Ashley Kumlien?" the woman on the other end of the line asked.

"This is she," I replied.

"Hi, my name is Cheryl, and I'm the executive director of the Montel Williams MS Foundation. We received your email about your run. Montel is very impressed."

I submitted the information on a whim through Montel's general contact form because why not? He was an Emmy-winning daytime talk show host living with MS, and I thought he would want to know that I was going to raise half a million dollars for a cure.

"Ashley," Montel said the next day, "it's amazing what you're doing. Running across America, girl? Are you serious?"

I was, and it happened that so was he. Montel secured the sponsorship to cover the cost of the run and flew me to Los Angeles to promote the event on a daytime talk show. I smiled, standing in the TSA line after appearing on national television, pleased with everything that had happened since Barcelona. The training, the motorhome, the sponsorship—it was all coming together. So I nodded in affirmation when the man standing behind me struck up a conversation and happened to be a photographer. I had been looking for a volunteer media specialist willing to come along, and there he was.

"These lines never get easier, do they?" the dark-haired gentleman behind me stated.

"I don't mind," I replied, floating in my thoughts.

"I suppose you just get used to it if you travel often. What are you doing in LA?" he asked.

I eagerly shared all the details—the cross-country run for my mother, my supportive boyfriend, the celebrity sponsorship, the feature on national television.

"I start at the Golden Gate Bridge next month," I declared.

Spade had an eclectic persona. His shaggy hair jutted out from a tweed paperboy cap, framing his friendly eyes and unkempt goatee. His leather messenger bag was chock-full of portfolios from his recent shoots—working with a gun-slinging cowgirl, then up into Alaska among the native tribes. He preferred to travel and shoot on the go, and he hadn't booked his next gig yet. My run fascinated him.

Before heading to his gate, he turned to me and asked, "Would it be okay if I came to meet your mom?"

Perfect.

A week later, Nate didn't agree.

"It doesn't seem right," he said in hushed tones across the kitchen island at me while Spade slept in the basement, having arrived on a red-eye into Milwaukee the night before.

It was just weeks before we would leave for California, and I was cramming a lot into the final month—a motorhome that we didn't really know how to use was getting serviced, then wrapped with the charity's logo. There was just enough time to pick it up, throw our things in it, and start the drive. A celebrity and a sponsor were in support of a nonprofit that was founded on the concept of me running 125 consecutive marathons, a feat that Nate insisted I come to grips with, which I still felt, after all the training, would be no problem. And now there was a stranger I met in a TSA line who I invited to meet my family. Spade had flown into Milwaukee to meet my mother and shoot promotional photos for the event. It was 11:00 a.m. the next morning, and Spade had yet to emerge from the bedroom.

"It's fine, Nate." I hushed back. "He paid his own way here. What do you want me to do? You want me to wake him? Say, 'Thanks for volunteering to take photos, but it's time to get up'?"

He turned his head to look over his shoulder, then back at me. "I just don't like it."

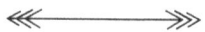

OF COURSE, HE DIDN'T like it. Another man would be joining us on our exotic cross-country adventure turned charity locomotive, neither of us acknowledging the force that now swept us along. Sitting in the motorhome together now, Nate and Spade sipped their morning coffee at the dinette while I sat on the futon couch (also Spade's bed), bouncing my foot anxiously, trying not to be rude, but it was after 9:00 a.m. and we really needed to get moving so I could run.

"Really, there's no rush. You have all day to run," they both agreed the night before. Knowing they felt this way, I tried to accommodate, agreeing to ease into the morning. This was their life too, and, really, we were just getting settled. Yet it was clear to me on this first morning together that their definition of "ease into the day" differed from mine.

Their steaming mugs of brew sat on the table while they browsed their computers. They'd take a small sip, set the cup down, then scroll some more. All the while, the miles crawled across my skin like an itch I was asked to ignore. *You have all day.* I coached myself, the anxiety mounting with intensity each minute. *It's okay. Let them have their coffee.*

I didn't want to seem crazy, being the only distance runner in the group, but the waiting slowly gnawed at me. Each mile was a finite task that I must do—and there were twenty of them today. The longer we sat, the less I could ignore the jumpiness of doing nothing building inside of me. Finally, I couldn't take it anymore.

"Okay, what'd ya think?" I said at last. "Time to load up?"

"Yeah, okay," Spade said, not taking his eyes off his work. "Let me just brush my teeth and use the bathroom."

It was nearly 11:00 a.m. when I finally began running, having driven up the route to park the RV, deciding the animal shelter parking lot was the best option, the director coming out to meet us and inviting us in, me being the only one hesitant about taking a tour at that very moment.

"It'll be great for pictures," Spade said. "I can have them edited and online before the end of the day if we take some now."

So we toured—strolling the kennels, casually walking along, the guys both genuinely interested in the experience, while I likened myself to the caged animals barking behind the chain-link fence. They paced. They leaped. They panted. That was me inside until the moment Nate pulled the car to a stop at the park I finished at the day prior. I hurled myself from the vehicle as soon as I could.

"Okay, I'll see you in an hour or so, up near Highway 37," I said, taking off in a run.

You should have completed ten miles by now, I scolded myself.

Moving along by myself, I covered an easy three miles through San Rafael before taking my route onto a set of abandoned railroad tracks. By then, my shoulders had relaxed. The miles were underway. Relief.

Admittedly, the roads around San Pablo Bay weren't as easy to navigate as I had imagined. The waterways and undulating landscape meant a lot of narrow bridges and curving highways. The frontage roads along Highway 101 weaved this way, then that—none paralleling the throughway exactly as the ones did near my home.

Looking at my path on my phone, a thin gray line on Google Maps revealed itself as a set of train tracks that would take me directly to Highway 37. I would run those, I decided, something I had been doing all along in Wisconsin for agility training and amusement, not knowing that this was actually illegal. No one would reprimand me now, though these tracks I ran upon were plush and overgrown with vibrant, soft grass. Grungy homeless men sitting on their cardboard watched me as I passed. Above them, a pair of sneakers dangled from an overhead wire. The men cackled. I picked up the pace.

I ran, joyful and light, as I had the day before, now loaded with snacks and basking in the pleasantness of being alone. The canopy of trees I ran under varied—sometimes shading my path, other times opening to fields of grazing dairy cows. They mooed. My feet swooshed through the grass.

Occasionally, I came upon spots where rungs had gone completely missing in clusters, deteriorated, or fallen through over algae-covered ponds. Here, I leaped across, landing on the other side like nothing could stop me. Then, six miles later, Highway 37 did.

"You cannot run on that," Nate said at our meeting spot, where the tracks met the road I planned to run. A cement barricade divided the middle of a four-lane highway–vehicles whooshing past. The barricade was an obvious protection from likely death if someone veered.

"I know," I admitted. A semi roared by. It was a busy road, cars coming and going in both directions well above the suggested sixty-five-mile-per-hour limit.

"I checked the map. There aren't any direct side roads," he told me.

I had looked already as well. "I know."

"Did you really expect to run this?" He asked, concerned.

It wasn't that I expected to run *this*. It was that the highway looked different on Google Maps while viewing it on my laptop in my bedroom. I typed in "Golden Gate Bridge" and used the pedestrian feature to connect my starting point to Sacramento, the next major city along my route. I assumed that anything that wasn't an interstate would be runnable. Highways were highways, right?

Wrong. Highways could be just like interstates, I was learning–a fast, main throughway that was no place for a pedestrian, as CA-37 was teaching me now.

"From here, over the bridge, to this trailhead on the other side, it's about five miles. Why don't you get in? We'll drive you," Nate suggested.

"Um, no." The recommendation appalled me. "There will be no driving me along the route. I will only be running."

Searching Google Maps on my BlackBerry, every road took me further north or back south again, winding me in directions that didn't help me go east. Zooming in, I recognized a familiar gray line.

"Here." Pointing to my phone, I continued. "This is a set of train tracks that parallels the highway. I'll run along here, and you two meet me at these crossroads."

Nate sighed. "What if a train comes?"

"I'll hear it and get off the tracks."

"And what if there's no place to go?"

"Listen, I'm not going to run someplace I can't bail from, but I'm also not going to get in the car and drive. Let me just log a few miles along the tracks, and we'll see how it goes. The next crossroad is less than five miles away. I'll meet you there, and we can reevaluate."

"I don't know. It seems dangerous, babe. How about I bring the mountain bike and ride along with you?" Nate offered.

"You're going to bike on train tracks?" I asked, now questioning him, imagining the bike thumping over rungs and sharp lumps of ballast gravel.

"If you're going to run them, I'm coming with you."

I shrugged. "Suit yourself."

Upon the tracks, I focused on my footing as I had been, landing squarely on my forefoot every few planks, light and nimble. Like a dance, my body knew the steps, and my mind enjoyed the challenge. Nate, on the other hand, bumped along behind me and jostled over the gravel at a runner's pace.

A few miles in, he understood my questioning. "This is horrible. How are you running this?"

"Told you." I danced.

Five miles later, at the road crossing—ten miles into my day and halfway done—we dropped the bike, now with a flat tire, and continued together on foot. Instead of breaking for lunch and an afternoon rest as I had intended for the endeavor, I needed to continue on to make up for the slow morning. Having "all day to run" was a cute concept that I wondered how to address to Nate and Spade. I was thinking of just that when I noticed the tracks ahead abruptly disappear.

Peering over the edge of the last rung to an expanse of water thirty feet below, we stood on the tracks at the edge of a river. They were rusted and abandoned. The middle section of the track that would connect us to the other side was opened perpendicular to the ones we stood upon, allowing boats entry into the bay.

"What now?" Nate asked, standing at my side.

"Well, I guess we don't have to worry about a train coming," I joked.

"So." He paused. "Are you ready to get in the car yet?"

Looking around, I thought about what to do.

Just north of us, down a steep embankment, was a small road that wound back west, then north before going east again. It was a lollipop bubble of a way around the river that would add at least another seven miles. Less than ideal.

I stared at CA-37, cursing its magnitude. It towered high above the water—a concrete speedway that was most definitely more like an interstate.

Damn it. Why is it so fucking busy? The tops of cars, shown above the structured siding, sped across. At the bridge's footing, along a narrow pier, two men loaded their gear into an aluminum fishing boat. The sunlight sparkled off the water. I had an idea.

"Hi!" I waved at the fishermen while I walked down the pier wearing a bright pink running skirt. "My name is Ashley. I'm running across America from California to New York for my mom. She has multiple sclerosis, and I'm raising funds for a cure. I started yesterday at the Golden Gate Bridge," I said, handing them a business card.

"Hi," the man replied, reluctant, looking at the card.

"I know this sounds odd, but I've been running along these tracks, and now they've ended. Would you take us in your boat to that section on the other side? We can climb the ladder and continue along the tracks without me having to add a bunch of miles around the river."

He looked at me, then at the card again. "You're running across America?"

"Yeah. For my mom. She has multiple sclerosis. I'm raising five hundred thousand dollars for research," I repeated, pulling up the website on my phone. "She's the sweetest. Her name is Jill. I'm from Wisconsin." Midwest breed, surely, they could trust me.

"Um, sure, why not? Hop in."

Nate smiled at me while shaking his head. "You're crazy," he said softly. I smiled back. He had always thought me to be both ridiculous and endearing, and I had yet to disappoint.

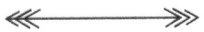

THAT NIGHT IN BED, emotionally and physically exhausted, I lay tucked under my blanket, acknowledging that this was a lot more than "just running" and wondering how to manage it all. It had been another sporadic day filled with unexpected delays—a slow morning, navigation discussions, parking issues, route changes, and, most important but time-consuming of all, connecting about the cause.

"I didn't tell you this, but my father has MS," the director at the animal shelter said to me when we arrived back at their parking lot for the motorhome.

My body was covered in a thin layer of dust and dried sweat. My hips were sore. Twenty-two miles of train track running were behind me—two more than expected for the day—and my calves told me how they felt about being light and nimble along the rungs. I needed dinner and a shower. A warm, cozy bed.

"He'd like to speak to you," she said with her phone in her hand. "If that's okay."

I pressed it to my ear.

"You're running across the country for MS, dear?" his voice said. "I went to your website. I've had the disease for thirty years, and, well, I can't much leave the couch anymore."

I thought of my own mother, how the disease cut her off, too, from the life she deserved, limiting her mobility and restricting her interactions. I thought of Montel and the first time we met. He told me how it was called a "secondary disease" based on outdated numbers of those diagnosed. That it lacked funding and research support because of it. That he put a gun to his head and almost took his life because he couldn't imagine living with the pain and misconception.

MS isn't a mortality disease, but it can certainly take your life. It's waking each day to the unknown of how bad it might get. It's the possibility of having unmanageable symptoms. It's the slow deterioration of mobility and independence. It's extreme fatigue. It's mental confusion. It's searing jolts of nerve pain. It's depression. And it's these things being invisible to everyone except those that know—a dire, isolating experience at times for everyone involved.

While I was promoting my event, people confused it with other diseases. "Is that that Jerry Lewis's telethon disease?" people would ask.

I'd vent about it later to my father. "People don't even know what this is. How can they care if they don't know about it?"

Awareness wove its way into my fabric. If they didn't know, I would tell them, and I was still figuring out what to say. My mother was no charity case.

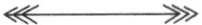

SEVEN DAYS PRIOR, ON a crisp Tuesday morning just after sunrise, we were in Wisconsin surrounded by an intimate group of new supporters—MS Society representatives, a reporter, family with extended friends I had just met, all gathered in my parents' driveway before Nate and I would drive 2,143 miles to my start. I hadn't thought to invite anyone, but these few asked what time I'd be leaving. It was exciting and awkward—to be leaving for my start, and also to be saying goodbye to my mother while they watched.

"I love you and am so proud of you," she said through damp eyes, her arms wrapped around my waist. I towered seven inches above her. She felt small, like a child.

"Come on, Mom," I whispered, steeling myself. "I haven't started running yet."

I moved from her embrace, and moments later, my mother lost her balance on the uneven ground—something that happened on occasion because of her MS. She tumbled before anyone could catch her and went headfirst into the motorhome wheel well.

"Mom!" We rushed to her side, my father being the first one there. "Are you okay?"

"Yes," she said, rubbing her head, embarrassed. "I'm fine. I'm okay."

"Oh my. Jill. You poor thing," a woman said.

Poor thing? I thought, irritated. As a family, we had done this all before—lifting my mom after a fall, her hardly making a fuss, getting her to the hospital a day later after wondering about the swelling, finding that she needed a steel plate for a broken ankle after all. She was as tough as they come.

But these spectators were just getting acquainted with her strength, a force that had nothing to do with her physical being. My mother wasn't a poor thing at all. She was a fucking warrior.

"No, no, I'm okay." She smiled, getting up with my father's help. "Just a bump."

How could I explain this tenacity *and* inspire the compassion necessary to fundraise half a million dollars? It was a complexity I continued to wonder about long after the conversation with the director's father concluded.

"I just want to say thank you," he had said, crying in muffled sobs through the phone. Sometimes, strength looks like letting someone in. "At times, life with MS can feel hopeless, but I just know you'll raise all that money to help people like me."

Too exhausted to hide my feelings, I cried too.

CHAPTER SEVEN

Run On

AND SO I RAN.

It wasn't long before I rounded San Pablo Bay and entered Napa Valley, where the scenery here surprised me. Expecting picturesque vineyards like the ones in the brochures, instead, I ran past beaten-down estate driveways, dust-covered with dirt and gravel. A woman in an apron carried a woven basket across a yard. The fence was wiry and bent. The roadway was worn and cracked. Paint lines, chipped and faded.

I ran and received messages from a winery nearby, a place more like the ones in the brochures. I stopped to meet the manager and take a tour, and I kept running. I ran through Sacramento, staying at the college apartment lofts after being invited by the director, ate sushi with the students, and kept running. I stopped for an interview at the capital, running circles around the reporter live on camera as she requested, like a circus bear on a unicycle, and I kept running.

Already within the first week, my days were a mix of spontaneous socialization and solitude. The endeavor asked me to be both independently strong and also engaging. I had to push through five hours of solo running each day—through the empowering highs and challenging lows—and at the same time, be up for an emotional or captivating conversation at any moment.

Since leaving Wisconsin, I had packed and unpacked an overnight bag seven times—from my parents' house to the RV, from the RV to the Turners' guest bedroom and back again, from the RV to a gifted hotel room and back again, from the RV to the Sac State lofts and back again. By then, our things inside the motorhome were organized, and often at these stays I'd find myself hoofing it back to its quarters for an important item that got left behind—a toothbrush, a recovery shake, the camera's memory card—making each moment a metronome of tasks. It wore, but if the stay was free and gave me a chance to talk about MS, I peeled myself off the couch and put on a smile.

As it always had, the running anchored me. My hips ached, and my feet were sore, but I ran and was also renewed. There were meadows of lavender-colored wildflowers, a cluster of birthday balloons tied to a mailbox, a vintage locomotive memorialized by the road. The fields turned into hills, and the hills turned into mountains lavish with giant pines towering overhead. A babbling stream chattered to my right. The sunlight beamed through twilight clouds. A rainbow followed a storm. I felt small, running past these things, in awe of life happening beyond my own. It went on, I acknowledged, not needing me to be there or do anything, and this reassured me—that I, too, was significant, moving effortlessly toward something profound.

Later, after the day's running was complete, I'd sit with Spade in the motorhome parked in some highway pull-off, reviewing his work.

"This shot is epic," he said, captivated by the image he captured while lying in the dirt—belly to the gravel, camera pointing, hand cradling the lens as I ran past him, flanked by fields of luscious grass. "See how the colors contrast your form? And how the whole scene is centered by the road?"

I did see, which only further solidified what I already knew—that he was both passionate about his work and also good at it.

"Why'd you choose photography?" I asked, looking over his shoulder at his laptop, curious to know his answer.

"It just came to me. I picked up a camera one day and knew it was what my hands were made for. I can look down the lens and know exactly when I've captured the essence of a moment," he said, his two fingers pointing forward from his face with one eye closed like he was doing it now. I found it impossible not to appreciate a story like that.

He reminded me of my high school art teacher—not in form, but in essence. Mr. André was a stout man, unlike Spade, who walked around the halls with a cane and a limp.

"Here's what most people won't tell you," the teacher had said to me one afternoon while I pondered my future with a raw piece of charcoal in my hands. "Figure out what you love to do, then find out how to get paid for it."

Of what I loved to do, that was easy. The gym was a place where loads of weight and clothes drenched in sweat were the makings of an honest day's work. You'd enter, grind through the load, and always leave a better version than the one who arrived. It wasn't always about lifting more or running faster. It was about showing up and doing it, no matter what. It was for everyone, and it was measurable—qualities of fairness that pulled at me.

Spade had followed his love too. "Shooting your mother was easy," he said, looking at me from the bench seat. "She has a beautiful soul."

I thought of her just then. Sitting on the couch at home, watching Oprah as she always did at this time of day. It was most of what she could do on her own.

"Well, then," I said, "you'd better get back here quickly. We need your help telling her story."

Spade, unfortunately, was already leaving. There was a lingering contract that he couldn't get out of, so he planned a quick jump up to Alaska for another client, then would return for the rest of my run. He was headed to a place I dreamed about—a northern, glacial landscape I longed to explore. With his upcoming departure, I couldn't help but recall what I'd left behind.

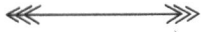

THE LONG RUN HOME

"**ARE YOU SURE YOU** want to leave *now*?" my ship supervisor asked. "It's the middle of the recession. Your run sounds amazing, but can it wait? Or could you train here? We're lucky to even have jobs right now."

She was right, of course. Eighteen months prior, the US housing market burst, creating a global financial crisis—a loss of $8 trillion that crippled the economy and wiped out more than 8.7 million American jobs. The country still teetered its way through staggering unemployment, and here I was with a whimsical reason to leave mine and start asking people for money.

"I'm going to raise $500,000 for MS research," I told her boldly, not even partially considering how the economy would affect such a thing. "I can't wait for something I can't control to get better. I just *know* it's what I'm supposed to do."

There was an air of mystery to the endeavor I knew I needed to trust—that if I waited for it to make sense, it never would. And, in truth, if I didn't leave now, I might never.

We had crossed the Atlantic, porting out of Miami for the winter, and the ship was headed to St. Maarten, Puerto Rico, and the Bahamas—places where creamy sand beaches met cerulean lapping waves. If I dared think about it, I could already feel myself warmed by the golden rays, heavy on a towel like a seal with a belly full of tacos and a joint to my lips. The smell of my skin toasted by the sun. Sand as fine as silk between my toes.

So, yes, I was sure I wanted to leave the ship as soon as possible, and, no, I couldn't stay in paradise to train, and, yes, I had thought about the economic crisis (though, really, I hadn't, but I didn't want to say that). My supervisor looked at me and nodded, then called headquarters for my replacement.

It was all very wonderful and romantic, bobbing around the ship for three weeks, waiting to go home, telling everyone that I was leaving to run across America for my mother.

That I was doing it for her was the raw truth I centered myself on each time my mind wandered to the pristine shoreline or the fear that lurked from doing such an outlandish thing. Families on vacation laughed as they entered the sports deck where I worked—parents dressed for a tan in their suits, pasty limbs poking out like starfish, corralling their children like a bunch of bouncing balls to the check-in desk.

I stood behind the counter, handing out waivers and smiling brightly at the same joke I heard a thousand times each day, that they were "signing their lives away." Their freedom to take such a lavish vacation, to climb a rock wall atop a cruise ship, fueled me like tinder on smoking wood—a parade of people who had what my family didn't. Mobility. Freedom.

More than that, though, my shipmates were like family. We lived and worked and played together, thousands of miles away from our actual families. Our months-long contracts kept on through birthdays, weddings, and holidays, and we found ways to celebrate together all the same.

My first holiday away from home, I snuck a six-foot Christmas tree into my cabin with my roommate—quite a feat with the port authorities scanning every item leaving and entering the ship. There were strict fire codes about decorations. We plotted and did it anyway, curious to see what would happen. Once inside, we erected that full-sized tree in our 120-square-foot space, adorning it with all the lights we could find. We mounted a fake fireplace with stockings on the wall and hung paper snowflakes from the ceiling. I imagine the safety officers, upon weekly cabin inspection, let our cabin pass out of sheer astonishment, like walking into Narnia from the wardrobe. Neither they nor we said anything about our cabin decor until after Christmas, when we received a failed inspection report and a note written in crimson capital letters: "LADIES, CHRISTMAS IS OVER!" We bent over laughing, then opened a bottle of wine, and dismantled the mischief.

I wanted to keep that job like nothing else, to travel to all the places around the world I imagined I would. But I couldn't. For what? To watch the fun unfold before me day after day? The pain of my mother's disease festering beneath the surface after the answer I had been given to mend the hurt I had run from all along?

I couldn't. So I packed my things from my cupboard-sized closet and walked down the gangway with my suitcases trailing behind me, smiling at my shipmates, hugging them, doing the thing I had told them I would.

And then I left, and the dream of doing it was replaced with actually doing it, and *that* was a lot less wonderful and romantic, with no paradise cruise ship and fascinated friends to bob around.

I sat in a stiff plastic airport chair after debarking the cruise ship for the last time, and the reality of what I had done dumped into my mind like a plaster ceiling caving in.

Run across the whole fucking width of America? Are you fucking crazy? I scolded myself. A stream of hot tears fell down my damp face, stifling my sobs through a fit of gasps. *Could you not just try a marathon first?* Now, doing that seemed like an obvious first step, but I had been too enthralled with the endeavor to even consider it on the ship. And I was gone now. Alone. Heading to Wisconsin in the dead of winter to move back into my childhood bedroom in my parents' junk-filled home. *Fucking great.*

Fear, I found, has a way of waiting for the opportune time to arrive.

Through my sobs, I heard the airport speaker call out–*First call for Flight 107, nonstop to Milwaukee.*

My neighbors began to rustle, tucking away their books, their laptops, stuffing the last bit of their coffee shop croissants into their mouths, crumpling up the translucent tissue, and wiping away the crumbs.

I dried my wet face with my shirt, absent of tissue because I hadn't thought I would cry, and took a deep breath. In an open journal on my lap, I did the only thing I could think to do–push away the insecurity with ink.

You can do this. I wrote, summoning the conviction I felt on the treadmill. *You can do this. You can do this.*

Standing, I handed over my boarding pass. "Going home or just visiting?" the attendant asked with a smile.

"Home," I replied, "I'm going home." Then I marched down the gangway and, like a bird, I migrated north to familiar land for the next year and thirty-seven days.

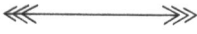

THAT FAMILIAR LAND WAS east of me now, and I was running to it on an incline.

Twenty-four miles east of Sacramento, a day after Spade departed in a cab, the elevation rose and wouldn't let up for the next five days. Running through Pollack Pines now, I was midway through this ninety-five-mile ascent, where I'd finally reach its precipice at the top of my first summit near Lake Tahoe. I knew none of these details—the distance of the incline nor its peak up ahead. Rather, just what my body told me—that my calves were sore, and they, along with my first blister, were tender to the touch.

Hours earlier, in preparation to run, I lanced that blister with a sewing needle on the futon couch where Spade had slept. I pushed the pointed metal into my skin and watched a teardrop of liquid ooze out of the hole. I pressed hard on the spot with a Kleenex, squeezing the blister dry but keeping the skin intact. I needed the extra protection to allow the fleshy pink underneath to toughen before tearing the dead flap of white skin away from my foot. I wrapped my blistered fourth toe in duct tape, a funny little phalange that was long and tucked in beneath my third toe, which is why it was blistering in the first place, then covered that with an athletic skin lubricant called Body Glide.

"Is that normal?" Nate asked, watching me carry out my foot care. "Are you supposed to use duct tape like that?"

I looked up at him, cradling my forefoot in my hands. "What's normal?" I said, pulling on my sock. "It works. That's all I care about."

Nate and I had had a relaxing morning, waking up for the first time in ten days without a nomadic photographer on the couch. Nate brewed his coffee shirtless, then sat with his warm cup of joe and stared out the dinette picture window at a forest of pines recently dusted with snow.

"This is nice," he said in his smooth Australian accent. I had to admit he was right.

Having a stranger sleep on the couch for six months wasn't something I had completely thought through, among other things. There was a reservedness that came with three newly acquainted adults sharing a tiny bathroom, kitchen, and living space (that also served as a bedroom), all within a couple hundred square feet. With him gone, I found our space more relaxed.

I stood at the refrigerator, a condensed version of the one you'd find in a home. It had a little black switch with a tiny green light located between the fridge and freezer doors. When that light blinked, we needed more propane, or the unit would stop cooling, and our food would turn to dank mush, a lesson we learned after sleeping at the Sac State apartment lofts for two nights and failing to check the gas. We cleared the soggy food into a garbage bin and started again.

Looking inside, I considered my options. A block of cheddar cheese, hummus, a carton of almond milk, red grapes, a dozen eggs, two chilled cans of ginger ale, and Greek yogurt. I grabbed the eggs and lit the stove burner.

With Spade returning somewhere in Nevada, I trusted that we'd adjust—me being willing to make it all work and them following along with. One year prior, a woman sailed the Lake Michigan perimeter on her own for charity. She was stalked online from her blog posts and assaulted on her boat. I had read the online article and thought about my own well-being, both undeterred and also hopeful I'd not end up alone pushing a stroller, as was my backup plan.

Studying Nate while he enjoyed his coffee, I wondered what his lengths were. Knowing my own, I realized that I had never asked him his. Before I thought to do so, we gathered our things, and I hit the incline.

Running along the frontage road that paralleled Highway 50, the shoulder was tight. I ran against traffic, eating up pavement well into the lane until a car appeared. Then I'd canter over to a shallow ditch blanketed with layers of reddened needles that dropped from above.

Just beyond the gully line, where the earth was soft beneath my feet, were modest bungalow homes with meager yards, and running past them, I envied their owners. My parents owned theirs, but still, it was shared walls—a caramel two-story townhome backed up against dense woods, located on a street named after my mother, Jill Court. The roads where I ran now were not people names; they were trees—Ponderosa, Evergreen, and Spruce. The air smelled, too, of these fresh, beautiful things.

RUN ON

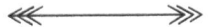

"**YOU'RE ON THE PONY** Express!" my father said to me via email. "This thing went all the way from Sacramento, through Salt Lake City, into Wyoming, and ends south of Omaha. Here's a link for some light reading. Keep an eye out for historical markers. You'll be on it quite a bit."

Not long after, there one was.

The historical marker was a bronzed medallion cemented into a river rock wall. On it, a horse galloped at great speed, hovering above the ground. Its mane and tail whipped behind it, the man upon its back leaning into the wind.

Running by it, I stopped in my tracks to read its inscription, recalling all the times I did this very thing at my father's side on various highways across the country, him being the kind of person who pulled the car over to read historical markers, making me subject to *this-happened-here* my whole life.

"This was the site of a popular roadhouse where the ponies of the Central Overland Pony Express were changed during July 1, 1860–June 30, 1861," the marker read. "From here, the route continues westward through Folsom and eastward through Rescue, Dry Creek Crossing, and Missouri Flat to Placerville."

I looked east toward Placerville, where I was headed—running a path that many only thought to do on horseback.

The Pleasant Grove House, marked by this plaque, had seen its better days. Its weathered white shingled siding hung off like tilted picture frames in whole sections on each side. Bushes around the perimeter were overgrown, casting dark shadows. Vines crawled up the front porch. It was the kind of place children dared each other to touch before scurrying away in fear. Once significant, its grandeur was noted and short-lived. Busyness and purpose turning to decay.

I snapped a picture to send to my father and to post on my photo blog, and continued running. Two days later, I found my own kind of marker.

"I got one!" I shouted out to Nate while walking toward the car. He had pulled off along Highway 50 in the only outcropping he could find for miles. By now, I was actually running on Highway 50, sandwiched between a mountain face on one side and a rivered ravine on the other. The subsidiary roads had all merged into a singular vein, making this the only passage between Pollack Pines and South Lake Tahoe. It was well-traveled and narrow. Nate questioned if it was safe. I tied on my shoes and kept running.

"That's great, babe. Let me see. What state is it?" he asked.

I handed him a tattered California license plate—personalized for RBEEG with a royal-blue heart.

"How cool is that?" I said, pining over it. It was the first license plate I found for the collection I planned to gather during my journey. I was hopeful to find one from each state.

"Very cool," he said. "I mean, honestly, when you told me you wanted to collect these, I didn't think we'd find any. But here it is!"

"Yup," I exclaimed. "We'll find them all over the place." I didn't bother to say that some would still be attached to their bumpers, ripped from the front of their vehicles—sometimes by the wind, sometimes by collision. Instead, I bit into a banana while Nate filled my water bottle. I had another ten miles along the winding mountain road before I'd be done for the day. As far as I could see, all of it looked to be uphill.

"Hi there," a woman called out, partially opening a covered patio door to a cedar-shingled restaurant where Nate had parked. The restaurant's fluorescent "Open" sign was off.

"Hi," Nate called back, raising his hand in the air.

"Can I help you?" she asked.

"We're all right," Nate called out, now walking toward the woman. "She's running across America. I'm helping her."

The woman stayed in the doorway, wrestling with what was her dog—an Akita, a massive Japanese guard dog that easily weighed a hundred pounds but looked to be well over that. Its fluffy coat was deceiving. Its height was intimidating.

"I'll come out, but I have a dog," she said. Just then, the Akita wiggled through, bounding toward Nate. "Don't worry," she shouted. "He's friendly."

Nate braced himself while the dog bounced and sniffed a circle around him, wagging its tail. He appeared to be friendly, as she said, but he was enormous all the same. I stepped forward to pet the big, happy fella.

"His name is Kazoo, and I'm Nancy," she said, reaching out her hand. "Now, what is it you kids are doing out here?"

Nancy was talkative and engaging. She had long brown hair, bangs that met just above her eyes, and two great big dimples, one in each cheek. Dante was her son, and she and her husband named their business after him—Dante's on the River—a waterside restaurant that had live-in quarters for the family up above.

"Well, you'll have to come back when you're done running for the day," she said after we talked for a bit, me still petting Kazoo, not needing to bend down to do so. "You'll be hungry, right?"

Hungry wasn't the half of it. When I ate now, I ate ravenously. I'd sit down at the motorhome's dinette to check my email in between runs and eat through calorie-packed creations of my own making. There were peanut-butter-and-jelly sandwiches with craisins and granola piled onto each goo-covered slice of bread. Whole bags of salt-and-vinegar chips disappeared. Plates filled with romaine leaves, grape tomatoes, feta cheese, kalamata olives, and hummus were devoured in minutes. I ate bananas, pasta with marinara chicken, falafel pita pockets, rice and beans, chocolate chip cookies, all the Subway, and I lived by two nutritional rules.

First, eat within thirty minutes after each run—an important rule for recovery during the optimal window when my body was a sponge for fuel. This would replenish depleted nutrients and prevent critical muscle mass breakdown. Ignoring this rule meant that muscle would be used for energy, opening my body up to chronic injury and, worse, kidney failure due to a toxic level of muscle proteins in my blood. I'd know if I reached this point because I'd find blood in my urine.

My second rule was less life-threatening. Eat anything I craved; my body would tell me what it needed.

Later that evening, Nancy placed a plate full of penne noodles covered with marinara tomato sauce and Parmesan cheese in front of me, alongside a basket full of buttered garlic bread.

"So, what's the plan for moving along?" she asked, pouring me a glass of red wine. "How do you pick where you stay?"

I looked eagerly at the drink, trying not to show it. As far as I was concerned, the whole point of drinking was to unwind, and I had no problem gulping the slight glass set before me in two or three swallows before another, more generous, glass would be poured if Nate and Nancy weren't here. Nate didn't have this same issue. I knew this by the way he put whole glasses of alcohol down for lengths of time while talking to people. He didn't cling to it in a crowd as I did, like a life vest.

"We're mostly looking for free spots. Wherever we're allowed to park the RV," I replied, the metal of my fork tapping the porcelain plate each time I stabbed a noodle. "The motorhome is fully sustainable on its own."

"I can't imagine that leaves a lot of options around here," Nancy stated.

"It hasn't been easy," Nate admitted. "Especially when we're looking for a free place. I feel like we're hobos, always intruding and expected to move along. We're parked over in Pollack Pines right now, but we'll have to drive back there tonight and move it to somewhere in Lake Tahoe in the morning."

Nancy leaned against the bar with her hands, considering the logistics of the event. The bar behind her was planked with dark wood from floor to ceiling, and the countertops were a burgundy red. A magician's statue popped out of the wall, pulling a rabbit from its hat, and framed poster memorabilia covered the rest of it. The vibe was '90's supper club meets tourist attraction, poorly lit and random.

"How often do you have to move?" she asked.

I shrugged. "Every two to three days. Each run puts us at least twenty miles further down the road. By the third or fourth day, depending on where we're parked, it makes for a really long drive to get to and from the route. Though I'd sleep next to the road if Nate would let me."

He shook his head. "That's because you're ridiculous," he teased.

I lifted the bread basket napkin and broke off a slice. "I'm efficient."

The lodging logistics were already a bit of an inside joke to downplay the stress it caused. I wanted to stay close to my finishes each day, and Nate wanted safety. I wanted to save money, parking at obscure locations that we didn't have to pay for, reading a book on the side of the road after a run because it cost nothing, while Nate rested in other, more modern ways.

"The RV park has cable, and they won't ask us to move," he reasoned.

"We're not paying for TV," I'd counter. "There are plenty of other free things to do."

I didn't hate TV, but the event budget concerned me, mainly because I made it up. During planning, a business professor suggested that I find a similar business model to my idea and use it as a framework, which sounded great, except no one was running across America as a business. I pulled out a calculator in my bedroom and wished up a number for 3,200 miles of driving, which would end up being only half of the miles we would cover, me forgetting to factor in the drive from Wisconsin to California for the start, and from New York to Wisconsin after the finish, and all the back and forth in between. And that was *before* we had two vehicles. I filled up the gas tank of the RV for the first time, and when the pump timed out before the tank was full, I knew that the $3,500 fuel budget I had guessed at wouldn't be enough.

"We have some friends in Lake Tahoe," Nancy said, taking my empty plate and scooping on more food. "Irie and Steve. They'd be happy to have you."

A free meal and a place to stay? That was all I needed.

"Now, do you know what you're up against? Have you even driven the mountain pass yet?" she asked.

I reached for the plate that she pushed back toward me, shaking my head no.

CHAPTER EIGHT
Big Water

HOW AM I NOT *dead yet?* I thought, pacing my bedroom at my parents' home one year prior on the eve of May 8, 2009.

I stared at a chart of miles, aid stations, and drop bag points on a website, calculating and recalculating running time and calories burned. A drop bag, I learned, was a personal pack that each runner could put together before an ultralong distance race, appropriately labeled with the correct aid station for the race officials to distribute. With my alarm already set for 3:00 a.m., I would awake early the next morning to run fifty miles in the Kettle Moraine National Forest. Or, at least that was the idea.

May 8 had arrived suddenly, and I felt unprepared. It had been six short weeks since I registered for the event in a post-marathon delirium when it felt like there'd be plenty of time to prepare.

"Why not do a few marathons first?" My father had suggested.

"Dad, I just ran twenty-six miles from the house. I'm not going to *pay* to do it when I can do it for free," I said, thinking only of the cost, not of what I'd gain.

What I wanted to do was called ultrarunning, and until I read Dean's book, Ultramarathon Man, I didn't even know it was a thing.

It most certainly was.

Technically speaking, ultrarunning is any footrace longer than the marathon distance, and it's been around for centuries. As a sport, it began in the '70s with a niche group of runners going farther than 26.2 miles on their own, mostly through the woods, self-supported without any of the marathon glitz. Then it gained mainstream interest around 1994.

It was raw and simple, and it suited me. Get your ass out to the forest and run. You have twelve hours to finish. That person over there ran here from their house as a warm-up. They live seven miles away. Now, go. A volunteer who was up at 1:00 a.m. is standing in the woods along the course waiting for you. They will give you soup. When you finish, you get a free beer.

Who *were* these people?

I hoped to find out after I sorted out this drop bag thing first.

I had to consider what I thought I might need nine miles into the race and put those supplies in my number one drop bag, which would be transported to aid station two, a checkpoint where volunteers would be standing with fluid, food, and encouragement. Proper nutrition was essential, and I was just learning about what my body could manage.

Okay, so, bag one has a Pedialyte, two Clif Shot Blocks, Hammer Endurolytes, and Perpetum powder, I said to myself, typing into my phone's calculator. *That's 465 calories, but the Perpetum I probably won't use yet within the first ninety minutes, so minus 260, but how many ounces of liquid is this? That seems like a lot. I think the book says something about digestion rate. Where was that information?*

These were all things suggested for ultrarunning on online forums or in *The Endurance Athlete's Guide to Nutrition*. In text, my body morphed from something simple I knew into a maze of delicate biology: "*Endurance exercise severely stresses your body and depletes your physical reserves.*" Severely? Really? "*Without a finely tailored fueling program, your body will lack the raw materials it needs for cellular energy production, waste product disposal, tissue repair and maintenance, muscle growth, disease prevention, climate adaptation, and other vital physiological functions.*"

Mine was not what one would consider a "finely tailored fueling program."

The mess of products I ordered was an effort to avoid a repeat of my impromptu marathon—the absolute crumbling of my being until my parents showed up with bananas—and the products had arrived just in time for me to unwrap them from their packaging and divvy them up into drop bags. An elevation profile just below the aid station chart squiggled up and down like an EKG, and my gut fluttered. The Ice Age Trail 50 was not a cutesy marathon from my parents' house around a lake. It was something else altogether.

Just before 6:00 a.m. the next morning, I stood by my parents near a heavily wooded parking lot.

"Okay, let's bring it in," a man shouted over the crowd of runners milling about. There were a couple hundred athletes—men and women, fanned out across a grassy clearing. A woman wearing a teal backpack, not needing this information, turned and ran to the bathroom.

"Confusion Corner," the man shouted. "It's a hairpin turn to the left about nine miles in. If you miss it, you're off course, and either you're running extra miles, or you're disqualified."

I'd have to guess how far nine miles was and hope to not miss it. Drawn to running by its simplicity, I didn't have a GPS watch. My gear wasn't sweat-wicking. My socks were cotton.

Huddled near my parents and trying to stay warm, I felt out of place in the gathering. Other runners wore tank tops and stood in groups of two and three. A woman threw her head back in a laugh at something that was said, interrupting the man, who was still speaking.

How are they so calm? I wondered. *Am I the only one who might puke?*

Then a pop gun sounded into the air, vibrating off towering pines, and the mob of runners funneled down a generous grassy path. I ran along with.

"So, what brings you to the trail?" a middle-aged gentleman to my left asked after the lead runners dispersed forward.

"This is training," I said reluctantly, an embarrassing statement if I couldn't finish the race. "I'm running across America next year."

"You're running across America?" a different middle-aged man said from behind. Apparently, there were a lot of middle-aged men running through the woods. "What are you? Twelve?"

A few of his buddies chuckled.

"Don't mind him," the first man said. "He's vulgar."

"Oh, come on, Darren!" the vulgar one said. "I'm just having a little fun. It's okay, dear. I'm just having a little fun."

I thought of a note I had taped to my dresser mirror the night before—a reminder I wrote to myself amid the anxiety that bubbled over nutrition and drop bags. It was scribbled in black Sharpie on cream paper lined with ivy, a relic found in my desk from years past. It said: *You Can. Stay Strong. Be Tough.*

I was not this man's dear. I was nobody's dear. And having remembered that my body knew what to do now that I was running, I picked up the pace and left them behind.

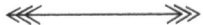

THAT SAME AFFIRMING NOTE was with me now, taped inside the motorhome's closet where I pulled my running clothes from each morning, among other bits of tangible wisdom—a law of attraction mantra, an inspiring magazine clipping, a telling poem written for me titled "Adrift" that had nothing to do with me being loose in the world, but rather how I'd discover myself along the way. These things were daily reminders, declaring me to myself each time I saw them. Reminding me of what I continued to unearth—that everything I needed, I already had.

Driving the Echo Summit Pass along Highway 50 with these things, I felt them to be true, even here. I sized up the incline that Nancy had urged me to prepare for—the narrow shoulder, the rocky vertical face, the guard rail that hindered travelers from the cascading earth on the other side—and felt calm, as if I'd throw my head back in a laugh if something funny were to be said.

I was alone, though, me in the motorhome and Nate in the Camry behind, up the mountain path I'd run and down the other side, on our way to Steve's house by way of Nancy's introduction.

Upon arriving in Lake Tahoe, I pulled into the gas station. All at once, a thunderous crack boomed within the motorhome, followed by the sound of weighted metal dragging across cement. The shocking and deafening noise made me think I'd been hit, that the back half of the vehicle had been torn away, that a whole section of the floor would be missing.

That's the moment I understood why people didn't loan twenty-five-year-olds their motorhomes.

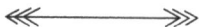

"**WE'RE IN LAKE TAHOE** now," I told my dad an hour later over the phone. "We'll have to wait for the weather to pass. The news says it might be a day or so."

I stood inside the Chevron Service Station and watched sleet pelt the window, then slide down the glass and accumulate on the ground. In the hour's time that we spent inside after finding that I snapped the spare tire hitch under the vehicle's carriage, the sky had turned from bright to gray to angry.

Nate sat on a stiff, plastic chair, staring at the winter weather advisory scrolling across the lobby TV. On a clear day, the mountain pass was a dangerous place to run, and now with a storm advisory, I had no choice but to set aside the ten miles I had yet to run for the day.

That's how Nate and I found ourselves on a chairlift the next morning at the Sierra-At-Tahoe Mountain Resort with snowboards strapped to our feet. The sleet turned to snow and fell steadily from the sky like fluffy white feathers floating from the heavens.

"We're taking the day off work to ride," Steve said of himself and Irie after we settled into their place. "Do you snowboard?"

Slope after slope, we dove down the mountain. I'd hit the center of a run, feeling a rush in my stomach and the wind against my face before cutting hard to the pines. I heard my board scrape against the snow, a slicing of the metal edge against fluffy flakes, and was reminded of the riding I did while living in Colorado. I spread my arms out wide, emerging from the trees and flying down the mountain, hollering in delight.

"Want a picture for the blog?" Nate asked, sliding in behind me at the lift.

"Probably not," I said, shaking my head no. "I don't want anyone concerned about my commitment to the run."

"You think that'd worry people?"

"I'm not sure," I replied, scooting forward on my board. "But I'm not interested in posting to find out."

There was the run, and then there was my personal life, which felt oddly mixed in some ways and completely separate in others. I talked publicly about my mother, my family, and running—these things being up for discussion—but they weren't the whole of me. I wanted to snowboard because I liked to, or bring my boyfriend across America, because it sounded like a fun adventure without having to explain myself, though I still did, people always having something to say.

The group in front of us at the chair lift slid forward. A green cage glided past, then swallowed them up from the ground. A single bar ascended down from overhead, loosely holding them in place from the fifty-foot fall that waited near the top. We were next.

Up in the chairlift, a horizon of white-capped ridges emerged in every direction. The sun beamed, both brightly from above and up from the snow below, and we had nowhere to be but here.

"What'd ya think of this?" I asked, looking across a snow-covered forest of evergreens.

"The winter'll take some getting used to, but stuff like this helps," he said, grabbing my hand, a gesture more than an embrace with our thick winter gloves between us like oven mitts. "Can we find a place near the mountains *and* the beach?"

"Sure! Why not?" I replied, optimistic about where we'd live after the run, imagining a place that would blend both of what we loved. "We can do anything we want."

He smiled. "Today's been perfect. Just what we needed."

What we needed was a break, and that's what this was. Fourteen days had passed since the start, me averaging eighteen miles per day of running since then, and the logistics of what we were doing had settled in mightily.

Some things were consistent. We knew it'd take me two and a half hours to run fifteen miles. We knew that to do that, Nate would drive up the road three or four miles, find a safe place to park, then either sit and wait for me to arrive or pull down the bike from the roof rack, clip on the tire, and ride back to coast with me. We knew I liked to get up early (like 5:00 a.m. early), and Nate did not, that ten dollars spent at Subway would fill me, and that I could sleep wherever there was a bed, except if that bed was near a light, mainly Nate's computer screen aglow next to me while I tried to fall asleep and he tried to catch up on football stats.

We knew that I, too, had obnoxious tendencies that bothered him, like that I licked peanut butter from the knife. Nate was so taken aback the first time he saw me do it that he scolded me like a child. I simply looked at him and licked it again.

There was the getting of gas, buying of food, restocking of supplies, cooking and cleaning, dumping the holding tanks, filling up the freshwater tank, and laundry. Lots of laundry.

Then there were the things we could never know. The heater could quit on a chilly mountain evening, the CO_2 sensor could alarm at 2:00 a.m., the water pressure could suck, a hose could leak, the radiator could break, and it all would. At a moment's notice, we were managing triage.

In the twenty days that had passed since we'd left Wisconsin, we had lived a lifetime. The day that I called my father from an Iowan wayside on the first day of our drive felt, quite literally, like many years ago.

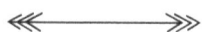

"DAD, I CAN'T GET the outlets to work," I said on the phone. I stood with the manual to the electrical system in my hands, one of the twelve manuals that told me how to operate the vehicle's systems.

Nate sat on the bench seat, looking at me, the other manuals strewn across the table in front of him.

We had read all the material—something about voltage differences and dry camping electrical use. There was a fuse box under the bed, a generator outside, and the engine battery that was different from the house battery, but either way, I hardly liked the idea of jumping the battery if that's what was needed. Each time I clipped the cables to a dead car, I was sure I'd electrocute myself, though I wasn't positive if we even had jumper cables if we needed them.

I'd been given a tutorial by the friendly mechanic who handed me the keys when I picked up the RV—a quick forty-five-minute run-through of how it all worked. But for the life of me, I couldn't recall exactly what had been said, and this manual in my hands didn't seem to help.

"Okay, let me see what I can figure out," my father said before he hung up. He always knew what to do.

"I don't know. Let's just keep poking around." I shrugged at Nate. He was just as clueless as I.

We were parked at a rest stop with free Wi-Fi, but it was the bathrooms we needed. The one in the motorhome, along with all the water lines, was filled with pink antifreeze, it still being freezing outside and us not wanting to burst a waterline. Drops of bubble-gum-colored liquid dried in the sinks and shower, and we still didn't know how to flush them clean when the time to do that came. We knew how to turn the vehicle on and drive, which also ended up being a near disaster.

Fast-forward to Utah three days later, and Nate and I hunched down to view what the gas station mechanic spoke to us about. "Well, you see this here," the man said, pointing with his oil-stained finger to a grimy, rusted piece of metal that blended in with all the other grimy, rusted pieces of metal under the motorhome.

"This is a shock for this tire here. It helps give the vehicle a smooth ride, and these ones in front are completely busted. I bet they're factory-issued, old as dirt."

We nodded. They looked like it.

"Have you noticed the vehicle bouncing around while you're driving?"

I hadn't. But what did I have to compare it to? I assumed the springiness was a part of driving a thirty-foot motorhome down a highway at sixty-five miles per hour. It was like not knowing how to use the generator for boondocking, or that we could lock ourselves out by engaging the deadbolt with the keys still inside—that I'd have to climb in through a window five feet off the ground to break back in—or that the holding tanks should be emptied a certain way—the black tank first (that's the one that holds the shit) and then the gray one (to wash the shit from the hose with your soapy, dirty sink water).

We learned these things while experiencing them. Each day, something new. And now, we gave ourselves a break by riding down a mountain on a waxed carbon fiberboard.

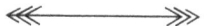

"**LET'S DO ONE LAST** run, then grab a beer at the lodge," Nate suggested.

I nodded in agreement.

At the top of the lift, an amber lager was on my mind when I slid off the chairlift to the top of a run. There, I sat in the snow to anchor my tail foot.

"Hey, let's go take a look at the map," he said, sliding in next to me. The snow crunched beneath his board.

I looked at my back. The map was uphill and way out of the way.

"We don't need the map. We've been here all day. The lodge is right there," I replied, pointing down the center of the main run. "Let's just take that."

"Come on," he pressed, "It's our last run. Let's make it a good one."

The mountain was small and beautiful, but the pathways were few. Plus, he had said "lodge" and "beer." I was already sitting next to a roaring fire, eating a burger, drinking a cold brew.

Nate marched up the hill, having already taken off his board.

"Ugh. Fine," I called out after, lying myself flat on the slope like a snow angel. I inhaled a deep breath, gazing up at a bright blue sky. Then I sat myself back up, unclipped my feet, and followed behind.

Standing before a massive wooden sign illustrated with colored clearings among clustered trees, I exaggerated my expressions.

"Here," I said, sweeping my arm in front of me. "Pick one. We've done 'em all."

Turning to find Nate, I nearly stumbled over him. He was directly behind me, down on one knee, smiling wide and reaching with nothing in his hands.

"Babe," he said, "will you marry me?"

My mouth spoke before I could think. "Are you... serious?" I questioned, unsure by the lack of ring, surprised that he was doing it so soon, taken aback that he was doing it at all during the run.

We had talked about marriage. It came up rather quickly in our relationship—being from different countries, leaving our jobs, and taking on this commitment together. We spoke gently through the phone for hours, him in Australia and me in Wisconsin, planning our future. We talked about the cost of him moving, about where we'd live, about a ring, and that's when I whispered back, missing him dearly.

"Nate, I don't need a ring, I just need us. I want you here."

When I said it, I meant it, imagining us as the kind of people who went on vacations instead of buying jewelry.

Still, alone and thinking of a proposal, I'd browsed the internet for rings, thinking he'd get one either way. *They're not that expensive*, I'd reasoned. *I'm sure he'll know to get a little something.*

I did the thing that people sometimes do when they say one thing to appear one way but then hope something altogether different happens. Like saying I didn't need flowers so that when he buys me flowers, it's because he wanted to buy them for me, not because I told him to.

And now he was here, kneeling in front of me just a few weeks into a six-month ultramarathon journey across America, doing exactly what we had talked about, and I was stunned.

"I'm serious. I want to marry you, babe!" he shouted, laughing a bit, giddy like a child.

I recovered, pulling him up for a hug. "Yes. Of course. Yes!"

He picked me up and squeezed tight, then brought his hands to my face for a kiss. I felt his heat against my cooled skin, his cozy lips pressed against mine.

"We're getting married," he said, looking deep into my eyes. "We're getting married!" he shouted to the mountain.

A few surprised strangers ahhed and clapped. My cheeks flushed at the attention.

"Let's go tell Steve and Irie at the lodge," he said.

"Okay," I said, smiling, following behind him.

Sitting down in the snow to ratchet on my board, I took it all in—the mountains, the adventurous afternoon, the proposal, being engaged. I was searching. To feel the way I imagined I would feel when I said yes to marriage—thrilled with my tummy aflutter like it was at the peak of a roller coaster. Below, Highway 50 cut a line through the ridges, the road I'd run as soon as I could, and I couldn't deny how disconnected I felt. The run was where I wished to be. It detached me.

Surely, if I weren't running across America, elated is exactly how I'd feel, I reassured myself.

My bindings click-click-clicked until my feet were bound.

"You ready?" Nate said, standing to ride, reaching to help me up.

"You lead," I said, smiling at my fiancé.

Then, riding down the mountain toward the lodge, I pushed away the feeling that bubbled up when I saw that the name of the slope we took was called Escape.

CHAPTER NINE

Snowcapped

THAT NIGHT AT STEVE'S place, I lay in bed watching moonlit shadows dance across the ceiling. This would be our last night here, and I crawled into bed early while Nate shared celebratory beers with Steve. I heard them crack open the drinks and clink glasses while I set my alarm for the morning. There was Echo Summit to run and an RV parked out front surrounded by a mound of snow. We'd have to dig it out.

Steve and Irie were an interesting pair—roommates, as far as I could tell. They rented a quaint Lake Tahoe home together near Highway 50 on a grid of streets crammed with a mix of log cabins and aluminum-siding dwellings. Rows of multiple cars were parked tightly on their snow-covered dirt driveways, and the place across the street had a Room For Rent sign in the window.

The trees were magnificent—giant pines towering above the power lines in every yard, making the homes seem smaller than they already were. It was the shadows of these pines that I looked at upon the ceiling now, branches and needles moving gently in the breeze, wondering nonsensically about the place across the street—what kind of room it was, living there as a wife, being a waitress and snowboard instructor in the great Sierra Nevada's, hiking its mountain trails every afternoon as I had done in Boulder. Until finally, I drifted off to sleep.

THE LONG RUN HOME

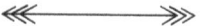

THE SIERRA NEVADAS ARE a spine of peaks along the eastern border of California that span approximately four hundred miles north to south, and a touch over seventy miles at its greatest width. Part of the Great Divide, it's a chain of mountains that links together from Central America, through North America, and up into Canada—a geographic separator of the Pacific and Atlantic watersheds.

There are the sediments on the western side, a gentle slope that trickles the annual snowmelt into the lush valleys that make up California's Central Valley toward the Pacific, where I had already been. And then there is the eastern side, a harsh escarpment that's cut ridged by a natural fault that created the range millions of years ago, weathered by wind, rain, and temperature variants, where I was headed.

In that direction, it could be unreasonably hot one day or layered with snow and ice the next. Its barren high desert into Nevada, where the Carson Range rose, would offer no breach against the force of winds that would whip across its land. In the weeks ahead, a local would tell me that the name Nevada meant "snowcapped," and I would furrow my brow in dumb curiosity, in no way having associated my former knowledge of Nevada with anything that would be considered capped with snow.

A mountain range is many things, I found, this one specifically having been formed millions of years ago by an uplift of granite deep underground. Its westward angles gave way to generous streams and massive collections of sediment while being home to diverse and beautiful forms—the giant sequoias, America's largest waterfall, and its biggest alpine lake, Lake Tahoe—known as "Big Water" by the natives.

Its sheer size explained the variation of what she offered, and most of what I learned of her was not her diversity or lightness but rather a cemented path laid upon her, twenty feet in width. And now, like the Great Divide of my run, it would separate the girl who ran with the help of her boyfriend to the west and the one who continued with her fiancé to the east.

The morning after Nate's proposal, I stood on that cemented path at the Strawberry Lodge on Highway 50, 8.7 miles from her 7,377-foot Echo Summit.

"I'm Allen," said the man, extending his hand, "Steve called in a favor, and I volunteered. My wife has MS."

Allen was a truck driver for the California Transportation Department, known as CalTrans. He wore a flannel button-up shirt and fitted sunglasses. His bedraggled hair and goatee were right companions to his weathered skin—a worn and reddened flesh that nearly matched his shirt. He was the kind of person who spent hours by himself in a truck, and this is what that looked like. Like my father—a man of the same vocation years ago when I was just learning how to walk—Allen reminded me of him, not in appearance but in circumstance: He was a truck driver, his wife had MS, and he'd wake up at 7:00 a.m. on a Saturday to help a young girl run a narrow mountain pass, expecting nothing in return.

"There are passing lanes part of the way up but not the whole way," he said with a comforting smile. "And I'll stay right behind you. Cars will either have to go around or wait." Then he turned to climb into his massive Mack truck with a snow plow fixed to its front. The warning lights flashed an orange glow.

I kneeled to the earth to tie my Gore-Tex running shoes, first tucking my windproof running mittens into my pockets before grabbing hold of the charcoal and fuchsia-colored laces. The upper of the shoe was made of waterproof, windproof, and breathable technology for chilly, wet weather such as this. They were stiff and durable, much like me, and would protect my feet (along with the wool socks I wore) from the winter road. My blistered-and-duct-taped fourth toe wiggled with the others to test the tightness of my tie.

The weather wasn't terribly harsh—a mild thirty-one degrees that I was well accustomed to from years of running through Wisconsin winters. Especially the most recent one when I sought out the harshest of days—running face-first into chilly headwinds, crunching through drifts of knee-high snow, lacing up during the lowest temperatures to callous myself for this very thing, to endure what came.

Even still, I had yet to learn how to halt the pendulum of my moods.

On a morning like this one, when I awoke with a desire to pull the comforter over my head and fall back into a nothingness sleep, the bulk of what I had to endure was that I couldn't.

Come on, Ashley, I commanded. *You know better. You get to do this.* My marching orders only making me feel more ungrateful. My mother would trade places with me, I already knew.

"I'll drive up along the pullouts and take some video," Nate said, standing next to me at the car. I slipped a reflective vest over my head. "You ready, fiancé?" He squeezed my shoulder.

"Of course," I replied, looking up the narrow, steep incline.

Allen and his buddies had done good work, making their salting rounds and clearing the road. The pass, now open and well-traveled, was lined by giant mounds of dingy, tossed snow. Cars rushing past made the hissing sound of tires across damp cement.

"I just don't feel like being out here," I admitted.

He gave me a half smile. "Eight-point-seven miles. Then we'll cozy up and rest."

I took a deep breath. I wasn't sure that's what I needed.

To the north of where we stood was Squaw Valley, the start of the famed Western States 100—a hundred-mile horse race turned ultramarathon foot race in 1974 when one of the riders, Gordy Ainsleigh, got the notion to do it on foot when his horse went lame.

"It was the most important thing in my life at the time," Gordy said of his younger self in an interview. "I just wanted to be a part of the experience." He showed up at the start on his own, gave them his name, and ran off into the woods. The very notion that he was by himself sounded divine—alone being a place I never minded being. My mind wandered from this show—a blinking snow plow to block traffic, a fiancé to film it—to a solitary fireplace where I wished to be in silence with a book and warm cup of green tea.

All right, let's go. My inner sergeant barked, pulling me back. *Drive your knees. Pump your arms.*

With a Mack truck at my back and a camera at my face, I ran up.

SNOWCAPPED

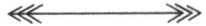

UP WAS A DIRECTION I trained myself to run—home being a place in Wisconsin called Lookout Hill. That caramel two-story townhome sat atop Glacier-formed rolling hills, up and down, waving through the prairie lands until the horizon met the sky.

In high school, I'd run from my renter's neighborhood down into an adjacent subdivision of single-family homes—colonials adorned with immaculate grass and heavy blooms—where I'd imagine a different life behind their doors.

Up I'd run, past the white one with a wrought iron fence around the pool, having friends over for a swim each summer. Down I'd go, past the navy one with the patio above the garage, or up past the chestnut one with the circular drive, or down past the taupe ranch with the American flag, thinking of a better existence we'd live inside, knowing all the reasons we'd never have one: They had mortgages, something my parents had long since paid off to make room for medical bills; they had steps, or a narrow entry, or a crooked drive, or... or... or...

My father meticulously evaluated all the obstacles that could arise living in a home not equipped to house the handicapped, if his wife declined, and she would.

It was tiring, all the mitigating, always considering the future that might not come. But what exactly did I imagine? That a single-family home would fix my father's hoarding? That it'd make my mother's disease disappear?

Still, I lusted for the homes, running up and down until I was exhausted and ready to climb the mound of earth back up Lookout Hill, where at its base, I'd force myself to sprint the half mile to our door, running so hard that my legs burned and my lungs screamed for air, until it was deafening, until it was the only thing at all.

Then, breathless at my parents' step, I'd drag myself back down. To do it again. And again. And again.

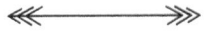

ECHO SUMMIT WAS NOT Lookout Hill, though, and I was not at home running from the pain. I was in the Sierra Nevada, fourteen days into a 190-day endeavor, running for it. So I coached myself up the summit.

Nice and steady, I told myself, lifting my knees as if I were running a flight of stairs. *You can do this. Mom climbs a mountain of pain every day.*

On the road, I let Steve do his work, blocking the cars from behind so I could focus on the run. I leaned forward, bringing my body over my toes and my center of gravity ahead. I dropped my arms, relaxing my shoulders and swinging long levers. I breathed out with force, pushing warm air out and pulling fresh air in. These were the things I knew how to do, controlling inward while cars sped past me to my left.

Up I went, working, pushing, and sweating. I registered the guardrail to my right. The hissing sound of tires on wet cement to my left. Nate at a pull-off with the camera. I noticed the sky—gray, and the snow—gray, and another line of cars—gray, red, and white. But mostly, I considered my mother, the real reason I was out here doing this ridiculous thing—running up a narrow mountain pass with a snow plow at my back on a day I'd rather be in bed.

Thinking of her attitude, her joy despite the disease, I ascended. She stood at five foot nothing, she could hardly walk down the driveway, and she was my fucking hero, a thought that brought tears welling in my eyes. It hadn't always been this way, me adoring her. I had been a teenager once—mean and disrespectful, and I recalled all the ways in which I made her feel less than—calling her "*only* a mom" whenever she tried to help, sighing heavily whenever she needed me.

"Mom, you *just* went to the bathroom before we left the house," I scolded her at a restaurant. "Why do you have to go again?"

"Honey," she'd say softly, "I just do."

"Fine," I'd huff, holding her stiffly under the arm to help her up. "Come on."

These memories surfaced, and, feeling embarrassed and regretful, I cried. *Why was I so angry at her?*

It wasn't until I decided to run for her that I learned of the vast disease symptoms and her sheer strength in spite of them.

She'd climb this mountain if she could, I reminded myself. And so I did too, thinking of her.

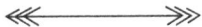

THAT AFTERNOON, BACK AT Steve's place for the last time, Nate uploaded the video he took of me running toward the summit guarded by the county plow. His commentary was bright and engaging, explaining why the plow was there, calling me brave, cheering me on. Sweeping the camera in a 360-degree view of the snowy mountain pass, the lens captured a bouldered cliffside, the narrow shoulder, the sudden drop off on the other side of the guardrail, and a steady stream of speeding cars that drove around. Only after watching it did I admit the dangers of doing it unprotected.

Settling in for a nap before digging out the RV, my email pinged with a new message.

You have a new YouTube comment, the subject line said.

"What a waste of taxpayers' dollars," a user wrote.

I threw the covers off and clamored down the stairs from the guest room.

"I thought you were napping?" Irie asked from the kitchen in the open cabin layout. A field stone wood-burning fireplace was the cozy focal point.

"I am. Some jerk wrote a comment on the video we uploaded to the nonprofit's YouTube channel," I said, walking to join Nate and Steve at the kitchen table. "I'm going to delete it."

"What's it say?" Nate asked.

"That the plow protecting me is a waste of taxpayers' dollars."

"Oh!" Irie said from the kitchen, moving quickly toward me. "People can be so rude." She hugged my shoulders to reassure and comfort me. She was the kind of person I imagined anyone could be friends with. Her wild, unkempt brunette curls framed a lightly freckled face, completely clean of makeup, which only served to highlight her round, sage green eyes. A decade older than me, I'd have guessed we were about the same age, or at least we acted like it. She was carefree and happy. A lovable spirit.

"I know," I replied, giving her a smile and hugging her back. "I'm okay."

"You are? The comment doesn't bother you?" she asked. "I couldn't imagine doing something so... personal and public."

"I mean, it's worth it for my mother. But I kind of expected this," I said, booting up my laptop, a compact MacBook that I bought at the Apple store in Denver. It was my first pricey purchase after paying rent that first month, after counting the cash from my new waitressing gig and realizing how much extra there'd be. The cover was layered with stickers I had collected over the years—a black-and-white oval sticker that said "Ultra," with a "Live The Dream" rectangle and a snowboarder catching air over "Life Is Good."

"You did?" Nate asked, looking at me curiously. "Why would you expect a comment like that?"

"I followed a girl running across America for charity last year and saw some negative comments about her online, which I thought really sucked. So I decided to read all the one-star reviews of my favorite authors and pretended they were about me." I explained. "After a while. I didn't seem to care."

"You did?" Nate said again, repeating himself.

At the time, the rude comments about the other woman's run really bothered me. She ran for something different, but still, I wanted her to do well. She threw a mattress in the back of a passenger van and had her friends rotate driving. She screwed a toilet seat to the top of a five-gallon bucket and took a picture of it for the internet. She stopped at charity events and spoke to young girls along the way. She ran across the country and raised thousands of dollars in the process.

"Isn't the charity just a feel-good way of running across America for yourself?" one person commented on her post.

"What the fuck?" I said aloud when I read it, offended because my run was no different, mad that people might think I was using my mother to fund an adventure, conflicted by the notion that doing something for charity meant there could be nothing for myself.

SNOWCAPPED

My mind argued with itself for far too long, reasoning all the ways I was a kind person doing a good thing for the right reasons. Could I post something about the importance of my why on the website? Write it into the copy so people would understand? How self-sacrificing did I need to be—having already quit my job, moved in with my parents, and founded a charity with no intention of paying myself—to make the reward I would receive, the accolade of running across America, acceptable?

That's when I accepted a truth that I was still growing into—that charity work didn't save me from criticism, that, in fact, in many ways, it'd subject me to more of it. Sitting at Steve and Irie's kitchen table, I had already started the ongoing, challenging task of accepting myself more than I accepted others' perception of me.

There you are, I thought when the comment hit my inbox. I erased it and moved on across my first state line.

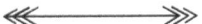

RUNNING INTO NEVADA THROUGH downtown Lake Tahoe, I came upon three towering casinos at once—Harvey's, Hard Rock, and Montbleu Resort. I looked up and ran past, wondering if Nate would work at one, wondering if we'd come back after I finished in New York.

Beyond them, the noble pines and snowy boulders appeared again as they had been along my route for the past week, unfazed by the boundaries of a state line. I was in Nevada now, but it all seemed the same as it had. For the next ten miles, I'd pull myself from the crummy mood that had emerged when we dug out the motorhome, finally, from the four feet of snow that had piled upon its sides by the local plows while we slept. I borrowed a snow shovel from Steve and went at it with the same enthusiasm as a chained prisoner.

Our bags were packed and tossed inside her chilly core when Steve pointed out the obvious. "Didn't you leave the heat on?" he asked.

We had not.

Upon arriving three days prior, with sleet pelting and snow in the forecast, we bound out of her and locked the door behind us, rushing into Steve's cozy home while temperatures outside dropped below freezing, not once considering that the vehicle's water pipes could freeze. Another day, another lesson of what not to do.

Inside, I looked at the wilted and cold inch plants on the dash and wondered if they were dead. I had potted them before I left—they were cut-offs from my father's plethora of greenery that he placed in empty containers of cottage cheese or whatever else he could find.

"Here," he had said, handing me a bundle of dripping stems with fresh roots dangling underneath. "Live plants are good for oxygen."

He was messy and thoughtful.

At least he could care for a simple plant, I thought, feeling mad at myself for not leaving the heat on.

Next, we had to drive the motorhome forty miles ahead to the Dayton RV Park across the state line, where we booked a two-night stay. Doing so meant I was leaving Tahoe and the mountains behind, or so I thought. I sighed and threw snow, missing the mountains already, not knowing about the Carson Range that stretched across Nevada and not thinking about the Wasatch Range in Utah—not knowing I'd be running over mountains for the next seven weeks, clear into June.

Finally, on the road running out of town after doing the necessary nonrunning things, I ran against traffic, catching glimpses of the clear turquoise water of Lake Tahoe through the peaks of trees. Around a long arching road, a whole clearing came, and I stopped to look. The stillness felt nourishing, and I inhaled. Moving on, I ran through Cave Rock—the rugged remains of a prehistoric volcano that was cut straight through by two half-dome tunnels that were Highway 50, twenty-one feet in height. They were the entering and exiting passages to and from Tahoe on its east side, and striding at ease, I let the earth swallow me whole and spit me out to what lay beyond.

Four days later, I realized I had nothing to be grumpy about, marveling at another Nevadan twilight sky. There was no one out here, made obvious by the highway signs that indicated no service for the next hundred miles. I ran marathons down the center of the road, and Nate and I settled into a solitude I didn't know I needed—until it arrived.

"Can you believe this place?" I asked Nate near the end of another day of running. I was at the car, plunging my hand into a three-pound bag of trail mix, crunching the salty sweetness around in my mouth.

Earlier that afternoon, I had run past a giant cottonwood tree rooted in a ravine, adorned with hundreds and hundreds of shoes. Shoes. Hung over a skeleton tree. In the middle of nowhere. I stood before it, amazed, as I did now at the setting sun. Every hue imaginable spread across a clear, unobstructed sky—blush, blending into sherbet, into lavender, into turquoise. Three miles remained before I was done, and I'd run it all in awe.

The desert is a revealing place, I quickly discovered. It's open and bare, being both terribly hot and bone-shakingly cool all in the same day. Harsh and arid, it doesn't pretend to be something it's not, simply not having the capacity to do so. Running along the highway, thinking about what it meant to be a desert, I found this place to be both captivating and beautiful—that what remained here is such because it has a compelling resiliency about it. That what's left to discover in this landscape are the things that are durable enough to be, and seem they always will. Like the coming and the going of a rising and setting sun.

"It is beautiful," Nate agreed, looking at the sky. "Did I ever tell you that, the last time I was in Nevada, I spent three grand in one night on drinks at the Bellagio in Vegas?"

"Three grand on drinks!" I gawked.

He raised his eyebrows and nodded his head.

"Why?"

"Why not?" He shrugged. "I was with some mates from the ship in between contracts, and I had always wanted to go. We got a room at the Bellagio and went all out. It wasn't all for me," he said. "I'd buy some. They'd buy some. We'd buy some for the women we were talking to."

"Three grand, though," I said, shaking my head and crunching trail mix. "I just can't imagine spending that much on drinks in one night."

"You never had to." He smiled. "You were milking 'em off suckers like me."

I laughed. "Fair enough."

"Hey." He paused. "Why haven't you posted anything about our engagement yet?"

My brow crinkled. "What do you mean? We called my family, my friends. Everyone knows."

"Yeah, but you haven't written a blog or anything about it."

"The blog's about the event. I'm not going to post a personal story about you and me on the charity's blog," I explained.

"What about your Facebook? That's not the charity's. You haven't posted anything there."

"Okay." I shrugged. "I'll write a post on Facebook."

Even after I said it, I could tell I didn't want to—something about people I didn't know following my posts because of the event made me feel like keeping some things private. But I could relate to what he was asking—validation of who we were as a couple, something I had done in college myself, waiting for a boyfriend to change his status to "In A Relationship With..." to declare our significance, not fully buying into the explanation that "a social media status didn't matter." I didn't want that questioning for Nate. I'd happily post about us. I changed the subject.

"Do you think we should move the RV forward before I run tomorrow? Or come back and do it after the morning miles?"

"I dunno." He sighed. "Probably after you run your morning miles. How far of a drive will that be?"

"I'm thinking close to two hours at least, driving back to get it and then forward to Austin, plus tear down and set up."

"I know. I was just trying not to think about it yet. It'd be a lot easier if we had a setup like everyone else, towing the car."

"We don't need to tow the car. Our setup is fine," I said. "We're not going to buy equipment just to make a forty-five-minute drive every three days more enjoyable."

SNOWCAPPED

Finished with the trail mix, I pushed the air out of the bag against my belly and pinched the seal together at the top.

"It'll save on gas too, babe," he pointed out. "We're burning through gas. No pun intended."

"I know," I said, setting the bag in the trunk. "We can talk about it later. I should get running." I grabbed my handheld water bottle. Nate closed the trunk with a thud. "Last three miles, then I'll be done."

"Sounds good," he said, opening the driver's side door. "Hey, put this on." He handed me a reflective vest. I grabbed it from his hand, pecking his lips with mine and taking off down the road.

Later at the motorhome, I stripped my sweaty clothes off and threw them on top of a heap of laundry, noting that we'd need to do wash soon. Standing next to the toilet in our four-foot-by-four-foot bathroom stall, I turned on the hot and cold plastic knobs in the shower. The water splattered a hollow sound against the tub's plastic shell, and I adjusted the settings until it was neither scalding nor freezing. The water pressure seemed good.

Stepping into the tub, I pulled the vinyl curtain shut and lifted the shower notch. The spray switched from the faucet to the shower head, a dinky little arm that was fixed at eye level–its height being a necessity due to space, the ceiling being just inches from my head. Turning my back to the water, I bent my knees and dipped my head under the spray, letting the fresh water run through my grimy hair first, then over my sweat-covered face and body. It was a measly shower, and I loved it.

By the end of each day, my hips were sore, my feet ached, and my skin was covered in a thin layer of dirt and salt. The fresh, warm water, no matter how it was delivered, washed it all away. Once I was good and rinsed, I turned the water off to save the holding tank from filling up, soaped my head and body, then washed the bubbles clean before grabbing a fluffy towel and stepping out.

Cycling the water, managing the cramped quarters, and ducking beneath a dinky shower head every day reminded me of the things I always loved about camping–like real camping, not the bougie camping they had us do in Girl Scouts, when they called it camping but then booked us girls in log cabins on a manicured horse farm and had us do arts and crafts all afternoon. I wanted to do the Boy Scout camping—in tents, building fires, hanging our food from the trees so the black bears wouldn't come. And I told my father this, begging him to bring me along when it was time to take my brother, and when that time came, somehow I was allowed to go. I crawled into a sleeping bag next to my father, smiling at the nylon green shelter, feeling tough and real, feeling those same things now.

At the kitchen dinette, Nate finished cooking us dinner.

"Thanks, babe," I said, sitting down in front of a plate of cooked chicken, wild rice, and vegetable medley. I picked up the fork and knife and sawed at the meat.

"Did the shower drain?" Nate asked.

"Yeah, but it's been a few days. You should probably dump the tanks before getting in."

At max capacity, the gray holding tank had nowhere to go except into the shower when it was full, bubbling the bits of soapy food water it collected from both the shower and kitchen sink into the shower's tub—a function we discovered a while back after washing the dishes, then driving to our next stop with grayish-brownish, murkyish water sloshing about in the shower basin.

"Want me to do it?" I offered.

"Nah, you're already clean," he said, stabbing a crinkle-cut carrot.

I was grateful not to have to do it, though I would have if he had said yes. After dinner, he stepped out the door into the night, around to the back side of the RV, where a detachable sewer hose, fifteen feet in length and the diameter of a grapefruit, snaked from our vehicle to a shit hole in the ground. Wearing a pair of plastic gloves, he pulled the handle for the black water tank first, releasing the door that held our toilet waste. Our crap rushed from the holding tank, through the hose, and into the ground. The smell of doing this is exactly as one would imagine, a pungent combination of rotten eggs and spoiled milk. Even the citrus-scented treatment tabs made specifically to mask the odor did little to do so against the days-old crap-slosh that collected in the tank.

Next, he pulled the handle for the gray water tank, flushing the liquid that collected from the kitchen sink, bathroom sink, and shower through the hose into the ground, rinsing the hose of the crap from the black tank with the soapy food water from the gray tank. In the morning, we'd unhook the hose and tuck it in a storage compartment along the driver's side of the vehicle—a space that would always smell faintly similar to the rotten-egg/spoiled-milk combination that absorbed from housing the hose we used to dump the tanks.

The next morning, a rooster sitting atop a mangled, wiry fence crowed me awake.

"A rooster." I stretched, rolling toward Nate. "Let's keep him."

"No," he mumbled. "No rooster."

I snuggled in close, spooning his shirtless back. "Maybe after coffee?"

"Maybe."

After a minute, I rolled out of bed. Our mornings had become a blur of the same:

> 6:00 a.m.: Harpsichord alarm (or today, rooster).
> 6:10 a.m.: Get dressed. Brush teeth.
> 6:30 a.m.: A bowl of oatmeal with a scoop of creamy peanut butter, topped with craisins. Green tea with honey.
> 6:45 a.m.: Route review on my BlackBerry.
> 7:00 a.m.: Out the door.
> 7:30–10:30 a.m.: Run thirteen to seventeen miles. Nate crewing in the car, or coasting along on the bike, moving the car every few miles after I stopped to eat salt-and-vinegar chips before continuing on.
> 11:00 a.m.: Drive back to the motor home. Eat all the food.
> Noon–4:00 p.m.: Do "other" event business—like move the RV, find parking, go grocery shopping, do laundry, fill the propane, get gas, write a blog, reply to emails, nap (always nap). Sight-see if there's something to see or if I have the energy, but likely just nap.

4:00–6:30 p.m.: Run five to nine miles. Nate, alone in the car in the middle of nowhere, moving the car every few miles after I stopped to eat bananas before continuing on.
7:00 p.m.: Drive back to the motor home. Eat all the food.
8:30–9:00 p.m.: Pass out.

Repeat for six days. Take the seventh day off. And by "off," I mean, do laundry, go grocery shopping, fill the propane, get gas, write a blog, reply to emails, nap (always nap). Sight-see if there's something to see or if I have the energy, but likely just nap. Today was my sixth day straight of running—twenty miles, twenty-one miles, twenty-six miles, twenty miles, twenty-four miles, twenty miles. Tomorrow was my day off.

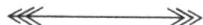

SITTING AT THE DINETTE, I lingered.

"Want to take a look at the route? Figure out where to stop before we move?" Nate said, sitting across from me.

"Maybe," I replied, cradling a warm cup of green tea between my hands. I stared out the picture window at a chilly, high-desert morning and tried to find the motivation to move. In the days since I'd crossed the border, I found myself sweating profusely in just a tank top and shorts one day, then layering up in two pairs of pants, a long-sleeved shirt, sweatshirt, hat, and mittens the next. Today was more like the latter. The wind pushed in hard gusts every so often against the broad side of the vehicle, swaying us slightly. A tiny whistle of air squeaked in through the window.

"What are you thinking?" he asked.

"I don't know. Nothing. Just trying to find the motivation to get out there," I said, knowing that motivation wasn't something to be found. The task had to be accomplished, motivated or not. Each day, the mileage counter reset anew, and I simply had to do it. Some days, that came easier than others. "Twenty miles just seems like a lot today."

"I've been thinking. What if I help?" He brought the coffee cup to his soft lips and took a drink. "I can run too. We can make it a relay."

"It's not a relay."

"I know. It didn't start out that way, but we can make it one," he said, leaning forward. "You can run the morning, and I'll run the afternoon, or we can trade off every five miles. You'll have more energy, and it'll make more time for fundraising."

I had started a social media campaign–Fundraiser Friday. Each week, I ran as much as I could on Friday, asking for a dollar for every mile. It brought in a couple hundred dollars here and there, tipping the event total to $31,000, but it wasn't the hundreds of thousands that I was running for. At least not yet.

"We're not relaying. I said I was going to run across America, and that's what I'm doing."

"Fine. Well, what if you do ten miles today and ten tomorrow? You won't get a full day off, but it might feel like we have more free time if you don't have to run in the afternoon both days," he offered.

"Holy shit!" I sat up. "That's it." Ten miles sounded like nothing in comparison to twenty. "That's a great idea, babe."

"Really? You like it?" He smiled.

"Yes! I mean, it won't give me a full day off, but two days of just ten miles seems so much easier."

"And then we won't have to fit all the laundry and shopping and logistics into one day," he said. "We can space it out a bit."

"Yes," I said again. "It's perfect. Let's just chill for a bit this morning and go out around ten. It'll only take me like an hour and a half to run ten today."

"Let's make brunch." He smiled.

I hopped up and went to the fridge. "What are you in the mood for?"

He stood and gave me a nudge. I nudged back and let him grab my face for a kiss. We embraced and didn't let go. In a moment, I knew exactly what he was in the mood for, something I hadn't had the energy to do since before we left Wisconsin.

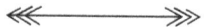

LATER, THOSE TEN MILES ended up being among a blistering wind beating at me for ninety minutes. I wore two layers of pants, long socks, a cotton T-shirt, a fleece pullover with a hood, and a thick, water-resistant powder-blue running jacket that had two ventilation zippers along each side. I left those closed.

After pulling my pixie hair into two spiky pigtails, I put on ear warmers and sports sunglasses that fit within the curves of my face. The sun wasn't shining, but I needed the glasses to protect my eyes from the grains of sand that whipped in the wind. They pelted against my face like miniature planets. I heard them *ting* off my eyewear. Within the first mile, I pulled my fleece hood up as well to protect the exposed skin on my neck.

Afterward, at the RV park, the aged woman behind the desk could hardly believe I ran through a windstorm.

"Is this considered a windstorm?" I asked, having never experienced one.

"Oh yes, honey," she said, shaking her head. She looked at me, concerned like a mother might look at a child. "Some gusts were upward of forty miles an hour."

"Hmm," I replied. "That explains a lot."

"There's more to come, dear. Y'all better hook up and hunker down. We've got snow coming and more wind."

"Thanks," I said, filling out the camping registration sheet she placed in front of me. "Hopefully, it's not too bad. Whatever I don't run tomorrow, I'll just have to make up the next day."

"Well, is it just you running? What about the gentleman with you?" she asked, looking out the window at Nate standing by our motorhome.

"That's my fiancé. He takes care of me while I run, moves the car up every few miles, gives me food."

"You're running, and he's just driving?" she said.

I looked at her for a moment, then looked down, and continued to fill in the form. "It's not just driving. There's a lot to do with an event like this."

She shook her head back and forth ever so slightly. "My husband would never allow an arrangement like that."

"He's not *allowing* anything to happen," I corrected her. "It's my event. He wants to help."

I knew this type of woman. I grew up knowing her. She reminded me of my crotchety grandmother–traditional and cynical. The same well-meaning woman who told me not to start a charity because it was "foolish," because there was "no money to be made in a career like that."

The woman at the desk brought me back to our conversation, "What are you doing this for again?"

"Multiple sclerosis," I replied. "MS. My mom was diagnosed before I was born. I'm running to raise money for research for a cure."

"Oh yes! That's that Jerry Lewis telethon fundraiser thing they do every year, right?" she said, taking my sheet and turning her attention to the vintage Macintosh computer that occupied a large area at the desk.

"No, it's not. Here," I replied, handing her my business card. "It's an autoimmune disease of the brain, spinal cord, and optic nerves. This is my website here." I pointed to the URL on my card.

"Oh, honey," she said, pushing my card back, "keep it for someone you meet up ahead. We don't have much to give."

"That's okay." I smiled. "I'm raising awareness too. You can read about it."

She reluctantly took back the card. I had the distinct feeling she'd throw it away the moment that I left.

"We've got a little church service in the chapel across the way at 9:00 a.m. tomorrow if you and your gentleman would like to join us."

I looked out the window at a plank-brown building across a plot of dirt and grass. Everything in the tiny town of Austin looked like a Wild West saloon. The people here were the praying type. I knew that before this conversation from the "Prayer Spoken Here" banner that hung seven feet across the camp's chain-link fence.

"Thanks," I replied, "we might!" Knowing that if we did, it'd partially be for event awareness and mainly because the weather was that bad. Since attending college, I rarely met with God in church, and when I did, it wasn't with the crotchety traditional type.

Outside, Nate and I set up camp in our spot—plugging in the electrical, attaching the water spigot, pulling on a pair of plastic gloves to attach the sewer hose before washing our hands, turning on the heat, starting up the water heater, and arranging all the items in the fridge and countertop that had toppled over in transit.

Just then, a massive diesel coach pulled into the campground, also decorated in a full vehicle wrap promoting a bike ride—"Brains On Bikes" was written in a bright-yellow thought bubble atop a light-blue background. A little black cartoon dog trailed behind a set of bicycles.

Even after finding out that Anne, in her midfifties, had brain cancer and that her trainer, Gundy, was with her biking across America for research, I couldn't help but feel a pang of envy. They had rolled into the campground like rockstars on tour—their top-of-the-line motorhome lowering to the ground on hydraulics. The two women descended from the stairs and relaxed at their picnic table, chatting with Nate and me while Anne's hired driver set up their rig.

"So, he stays with you then?" I asked.

"Oh no," Anne replied, petting the real-life version of the little black cartoon dog on her lap. "We put him up in a hotel at each stop. Only Gundy and I sleep in the coach."

We decided to have dinner together at a tiny place in town, and then I browsed her website before bed. A motion graphic of that tiny black cartoon dog chased two bicycles across the screen.

"It says her event is fully funded, though it doesn't say how," I said out loud to Nate. "I imagine maybe by her?"

"Does it say how much she's raised?" he asked, leaning over my shoulder.

Scrolling down, we both read in amazement—$1.2 million. Did I have to be dying to raise that kind of money?

The next day, I watched their figures shrink down a long stretch of highway while I ran. I had started earlier, being on foot, but they overcame me quickly on their bicycles and coasted briefly to say goodbye before moving on to stay warm amid the brisk wind that still whipped. The next ten miles, I ran, as I had the day before, bundled and beaten, wondering what it would be like to be her, the trainer.

Young, untethered, and into fitness like me, Gundy was riding across the country with her client for a cause in total luxury. It was the adventure in full without any of what weighed on me—the logistics and the charity and the donations.

She would die, of course, Anne would, battling a disease that few won, her own brain withering with tumors. But not Gundy. Gundy would go on, beyond the cancer and the pain, decorated as both accomplished and generous.

What a fantasy it became for me to leave this all behind and move on.

I would leave none of it behind, though, a thought that came to me as I wrote the organization's first gift for multiple sclerosis research, a sum of $8,000. My hand shook while penning the zeros in the charity's checkbook, and somehow, I knew that this would be my life.

"We're not even earning a living," Nate said after I shared how I felt. "How can this be what we do?"

"We have food, shelter, all these great sunrises," I offered, feeling a renewed sense of purpose. "What else do we need?"

"Income," he suggested. "An address. A plan for the future."

I said nothing.

I long since knew—from my mother, from Anne.

The future? It was a myth.

CHAPTER TEN

Edges

IT TOOK ME FOURTEEN days to run across California and eleven more than that to cross Nevada. By the time I arrived at Utah's border, I had settled in, having grown in ways I couldn't fully measure.

The things I could measure were the ways in which I now nimbled around our camper with ease—fully knowing its boondocking and camping systems, where to fill and drain the water, how to check and dump the tanks, the electric and gas functions of the refrigerator, AC unit, heat and stove, when to use the generator and how to troubleshoot a blown fuse. Full-time RVers, mostly retired folk, would stare, taken aback by my experience and confidence, curious about my branded rig, amused that I was as assured as they.

I knew how long it would take me to run each day (four to five hours), the gear that worked well and the things that I got wrong (the caffeine supplements a sponsor gave me accidentally taken as vitamins), which toes to duct tape (the fourth one), where to apply Bodyglide (my bra line), and how long it'd take to rotate ice packs (at least forty-five minutes). But also, essentially, those details didn't matter much because, overall, my body knew how to run.

I knew that Nate and I had our differences—that our sleep and wake-up times weren't the same, that his preference for relaxing was different from mine, that I was more comfortable running near cars than he hoped I'd be, and that none of that mattered because we were both out here to help people like my mom.

Mainly, I learned to ignore the concerns of those who had never been where I was headed. The questions of how it would be funded, where the RV would come from, who would crew me, how my body would hold up, and what to watch out for seemed more to be anxious questions rooted in a person's own limitations, which were not mine to own if I chose not to. Sure, my hips got sore, and my feet ached. My calves grew tender, and my toe blistered. My shoulders hunched over, and my stomach growled.

But I wasn't ruining my knees, nor was I aggressively aging my body, nor was I falling apart. All that was needed was a big meal and a good sleep to wake up feeling as fresh as the day I crossed the Golden Gate Bridge. My body was strengthened by the 661 miles that lay behind me, not weakened. So when these questions arose, which they continued to, I smiled and tucked myself away, shielding myself from ordinary thoughts that didn't fit my life.

Most of what I battled, though, was inside. When the sky was gray and the wind howled and snowflakes flurried from above, my mind cowered from the road back to the motorhome, cozy under a blanket. Still, I laced my shoes and ran.

What will I do when I get home? How would I make money? I laced my shoes and ran.

Why does my mind still yearn for a house even while I live this dream? I laced up my shoes and ran. Then, by no effort of my own, I'd wake up feeling grateful, and all would be pleasant.

How is this what I am doing? I would wonder, resting between the miles on the warm pavement like a desert lizard, eating from a hefty bag of trail mix. My mouth full of food. My skin warmed. My mind fully present. All was well.

These were the ups and downs I managed as my body did the same, submitting peak after peak across Nevada's "Loneliest Highway in America"–Highway 50, stretching over the peaks of Austin at 7,484 feet, Hickison at 6,546 feet, Pinto at 7,376 feet, Pancake at 6,517 feet (shortly after which, I ate pancakes), and Little Antelope at 7,438 feet.

Before crossing into Utah, I ran down my final peak and right into the town of Ely, where, after nearly twenty-five days of solitude with Nate, I was primed for something, anything. A cardboard sign stapled to a telephone post was made exactly for someone like me at a time like that—"Free Puppies."

"I don't know, babe," Nate said, shaking his head.

"Come on—let's just look. What else do we have to do? The dryer won't be done for another forty minutes," I said of our clothes being washed at the quiet town's laundry mat. "Pleeease."

Standing at the house listed on the sign—a single-wide mobile home tucked under a crisscross of power lines—I knocked on the front door. An overweight woman wearing a nightgown answered the door. It was nearly eleven a.m. This was the kind of place that would have free puppies.

"Hi!" I beamed, by now used to talking with anyone. "I saw your sign in town for free puppies. Can we take a look?"

I hoped they were in a pen somewhere outside. Instead, she ushered us through the front door and into a dingy living room. I stepped forward to a baby gate enclosure on the floor, ignoring the dim light from worn curtains drawn closed over the window, and picked up a tan fur ball with piercing blue eyes.

"A puppy! Nate!" I squealed quietly, hugging it, trying not to seem like we were for sure taking it with the bath-robed stranger standing right there. "What do you think?"

The woman made it easy. "If you'd like, you can take her for the day to see how it goes," she said. "You can always bring her back if it doesn't work out."

Nate looked at me and shrugged. "It's your run. I think you decide."

An hour later, we were at the pet store buying a leash, a squeaky toy, and food for the puppy we named Ely, just in case we kept her. *A puppy!* I thought, skipping through the store with her in my arms. She'll be our first child. *A fur baby. I'll run, and Nate will have a dog to play with for all the hours he's in the car waiting for me. It'll be perfect.*

The next day, while I ran five miles, it was not perfect.

"Ely shit in the back seat," Nate announced when I arrived at the car.

"Really?" I asked, crinkling my nose. Walking to the open door, I looked in at a spray of diarrhea across the upholstery. She didn't just shit a turd that we could pick up and toss out. She crapped a puddle of brown liquid squirt across tan fabric. The whole car smelled like our motorhome's rotten-egg/spoiled-milk shit hose.

"Damn," I said to Nate, stepping back from the open door, looking at the adorable fluff of fur in his arms. "Whelp, that was fun for a day. We're taking her back."

He looked at me and nodded. "You bet we are."

Forcing entertainment was hardly necessary, I realized. All I had to do was wait.

Four days later and 112 miles into Utah, minus one puppy, Spade sent me a message about his return. "Ash! Thursday is the day. Flying into SLC. If this is too late, let me know. I can rearrange."

I received the message on my BlackBerry while I sat across from Nate at a Subway. Of the few things I missed along Nevada's Loneliest Highway in America—strong Wi-Fi, movie theaters, and regular service stations—this took the top spot: a foot-long roasted chicken sandwich on Italian herbs and cheese bread, salt-and-vinegar chips, three-for-one-dollar chocolate chip cookies, and an iced Coca-Cola from the soda fountain.

"Spade's flying in on Thursday!" I said, pulling back the sandwich wrapper.

"Is he?" Nate said. "I wasn't sure if he'd actually make it back."

I shrugged. "He said weather's been a problem for their shoots. Plus, it's not like there's any place to fly into where we've been."

"True." Nate bit into his meatball sub. A drip of marinara plopped down from his sandwich. He moaned in delight. "This is *so* good. I missed this."

"You missed a lot more than Subway," I joked, equally enjoying our reintroduction into civilization.

"Well, there's nobody out there. It's crazy," he said. "It was just sagebrush and salt flats all the way to the horizon."

I nodded my head, agreeing. Not only was it desolate, but also every sign there was peppered with a spattering of bullet holes, which didn't necessarily concern me since we hardly saw anyone. "The sunsets over the mountains were amazing, though. You have to admit," I said. "And as a runner, it *was* perfect." No traffic to worry about. "But this is really nice too."

Into Utah, I stayed on Highway 50 and was almost to Highway 6, where I'd veer north. Here we found ourselves in the metropolitan town of Delta, Utah, population 3,436, a sign said, as I ran into the city limits. That was 3,432 more people than Nate and I had seen in the past couple weeks, and we were grateful for it.

Upon entering, the very first thing we came across was the Antelope Valley RV Park—a neat clearing of gravel and pavement that had a quaint cedar siding office, which was exactly what we needed because the motorhome's generator stopped working a few days prior and we didn't know what to do. Without it, we had no electricity unless we were plugged into an electrical outlet, something we managed to do by walking up the driveway of a desolate ranch, introducing ourselves to the homeowners, and asking if we could plug our vehicle into the side of their house. They obliged *and* cooked us dinner.

"So, what's the plan for getting Spade?" Nate asked. An overhead bell dinged in the sub shop, and a customer walked through the door.

"I'm going to have to do twenty-five miles each day for the next five days to get to Salt Lake City in time for the track club group. We'll be close enough by then to pick him up at the airport."

"I don't understand why you think you have to run up to Salt Lake City," he said. "Just run to Eureka, and I can drive you up. You're adding like seventy-five miles by running there."

"Nate, we've talked about this. I'm meeting with the running club and talking to three news stations. What'll they think if I don't actually run to their city?"

"Honestly? You're running across the whole entire country. I don't think they'll care."

He couldn't tell me anything, but he was right. I ran twenty-five miles back-to-back for five days, three of those days being additional miles, thinking it would be a whole thing when I arrived, thinking primetime news would cover my run, thinking the runners would be inspired, thinking that I'd finally see a spike in donations.

Instead, I stood awkwardly with the track club group on Saturday morning, telling them my story, and none of them had known I was coming. One news station didn't show, and the other two slotted me for another day. The most I saw of donations was a twenty-dollar bill and a two-page letter a woman handed me at an RV park, outlining the product she used to cure her autoimmune digestive disorder, along with a link to her site where I could order the product for my mother online. I folded the letter back together at its creases and tucked it back into its envelope, trying not to feel like shit.

Tacky product sales aside, the letter didn't say anything I didn't already know—that if my mother would eat nutrient-dense foods and cut down on processed junk, her body would, without a doubt, function better. Maybe even be rid of its chaotic, self-attacking disease altogether. But I'd be damned if I couldn't find a way to get my father to do it.

It had less to do with what he wanted her to eat and more to do with what he was capable of producing—how much more work could we ask of him for a result that may or may not come to be? When you spend every morning dressing your wife in elastic pants and Velcro shoes because, at the young age of forty-four, she can no longer fasten buttons or tie laces, you're not going to head to the kitchen and make a nine-ingredient, locally sourced, organic smoothie. You're just not. Not to mention all the other responsibilities weighing you down.

Instead, you're going to take the fucking five-dollar coupon that was mailed to your house, you're going to get in your car, and you're going to sit your way through the Arby's drive-through for a couple of cheap sandwiches because it's one less thing you have to do while you try not to cry.

I would not be buying her product for my mother. I would never even mention it. I crumpled up the letter and tied on my running shoes, then I ran toward Emigration Canyon so hard my legs burned.

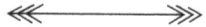

"ASH!" SPADE SHOUTED, THROWING his hands up. He stood next to his luggage at the Salt Lake City International Airport under a sign that said Arrivals, looking the same as he had–traveled, happy, with a paperboy news cap on his head.

"Spade! How are you? How was Alaska?" I popped out of the driver's seat and gave him a hug. It was good to have him back.

"It was great. Very snowy." He lifted his single piece of luggage into the trunk, and I pushed it closed. "It's good to be back, though. I'm so bummed I missed the engagement. I could have taken photos."

"*That* would have been amazing," I said, walking to the driver's door. "You'll have to blame Nate for that one."

In the car, Nate sat in the passenger seat, and Spade got in back. I shifted into drive and looked over my left shoulder, then pulled into airport traffic and onto I-80 toward the canyon.

"I'd like to squeeze in another five miles. Then we can settle in for the night," I said, giving Spade the rundown of the rest of the day.

"It doesn't even make sense," Nate grumbled, looking out the window.

"Nate," I replied, saying his name as a full sentence, like I didn't want him to start into it.

"What doesn't make sense?" Spade asked from the back.

"Ashley ran an extra seventy-five miles to Salt Lake City when she didn't have to. I want to drive that forward on the route, to drop her seventy-five miles ahead, and she insists on continuing from here," he explained.

"We're not driving forward on the route," I said.

"It's not cheating," Nate replied, raising his voice. "You already ran it."

"I'm running point to point," I stated. "That's it. That's the event."

"Spade, what do you think?" Nate asked, turning in his seat toward the back. "Do you consider that cheating?"

"It doesn't matter what Spade thinks," I said before Spade could answer. "When you run across America, I'll do it how you want.

This time, we do it my way. I'm not driving forward. Not for you. Not for Spade. Not for anyone."

I pulled the car into the parking lot along Emigration Canyon, the same spot where I'd left off from my last run. The RV was parked across a stretch of four parking spaces. Nate opened the door and got out. I turned in my seat toward Spade, feeling embarrassed that this was what he came back to.

"Sorry about that. I think he just needs a little space."

"Yeah, no worries," Spade replied, seeming completely at ease. "I know how it is. Crew can get at each other all the time on long shoots. It's a lot of work without much personal space."

"Right." I sat for a moment, considering that. "Well, how do you feel about crewing me in the car and Nate can have some space in the motorhome?"

"Sure," Spade said, patting his bulky backpack at his side. "I've got my camera equipment right here."

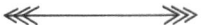

BEFORE RUNNING UP EMIGRATION Canyon, I stood before the This Is the Place Monument, a historical shrine for the Latter-Day Saints Church, believing themselves to be "the restoration of the original church of Jesus Christ." I considered this. The original church of Jesus? How many other churches considered themselves also to be the original?

I grew up in a strict Lutheran setting, attending the very same grade school and church my mother did through her youth. It was small and safe, regimented and consistent. Each January, every family member received fifty-two small envelopes bound together by perforated edges. Then, every Sunday, I sat on stiff wooden pews, drawing sunshine and flowers on my envelope with the tiny pencil that was stuck to the back of the pew in front of me, trying not to fall asleep. The envelopes were crisp and numbered to track my weekly tithe. I was eight. Was this worship?

In high school, a taste of something more vibrant came along with the introduction of my club soccer coach. He was competitive and encouraging, loud and honest. He'd yell hilarious forms of motivation from the sidelines each time the ball didn't quite get where it needed to.

"Almost, Ashley! Almost! That doesn't quite win games, though. Try again!"

Everyone on both sides of the field could hear, but somehow, it never felt degrading. It surprised me to find out that he was also a pastor. His church had chairs with cushions. Music was played with a drum set and electric guitars. The first time I attended, the songs vibrated within my chest. Now, *this* was worship.

In college, I couldn't help but wonder what I believed. Was my gay best friend really damned to hell because of who she loved, despite having a wonderful, caring heart? Why was it that some churches allowed female pastors and others didn't? Was I really to believe that God didn't make women to be spiritual leaders? Why were there varying standards depending on who was interpreting the text? And why did Christianity have as many colorful sects as there were leaders?

Who am I trusting? I'd think, listening to another male pastor interpret God for me. My mother was all-in, wearing "Jesus Is Risen" shirts like a walking billboard. What would he say if he rose now, I'd wonder—God arriving to witness all these confusing, conflicting, excluding rules that felt everything but loving.

Yet, running now, I felt a deep connection with God on this path that I was assigned. There had been many unknowns. There still were. Yet I felt safe. Guided. I stood at the This Is the Place Monument and wondered if that's how all these churches got started. That God made it that way so that there'd be as many ways to find him as there were people willing to heed a calling.

"All right, I'm all set," Spade said, coming up next to me at the monument.

"Okay, let's do this," I replied. "We're headed that way."

I pointed east, up Emigration Canyon.

Running the mountain ascent, I felt strong. After running thirty-five marathons in six weeks, my calves expanded with muscle, and my lungs breathed with increased strength. At the incline, I checked my form.

Lean forward, my commander coached, and I tilted my upper body forward—not a hunch of my shoulders, rather a tipping into the slope. Gravity pushed at my back, driving me up. *Relax your arms.* And they dropped, loose and intentional, beating back and forth like a drum. *Quick exhales—in,* out, *in,* out. And my breathing steadied. *High knees.* And my legs hiked, trotting up like a stallion. These details consumed me, graciously muting the growing burn within my chest and legs. That and the surrounding beauty.

Overhead, a hawk glided, peering down at me upon the road. I snaked this way and that in the cracks of the foothills, like a leaf upon a river moving through rocky crests. Up the incline, the car was parked to the side with its hazards flashing. Spade craned his head toward the sky to watch the bird, his camera in hand. *Click, click, click, click.*

The road cut a switchback, back the other way, then returned again. I was ascending, something I had been doing since I ran from the California coast. Salt Lake City sat at 4,226 feet, and I hardly even registered the air difference, acclimating to it day by day as I inched my way up in elevation.

I couldn't say the same about the RV generator. The trouble we had been having with it was an easy fix after all—an adjustment of the altimeter that controlled airflow to the engine.

"Why didn't it give us issues in Nevada?" I asked the mechanic. "I was at six thousand feet, give or take, the whole way."

He just shrugged at me. "It's working now, isn't it?" The engine hummed, and I wouldn't argue with that.

But it wasn't the generator that would cause trouble now. I drove myself up the mountain, while somewhere else along I-80, the motorhome had all but exhausted its ability to drive up. The heat gauge shot to red, and steam poured from the hood. Nate pulled the vehicle over and killed the engine.

My BlackBerry buzzed: "Babe, it's the RV. We've got a problem."

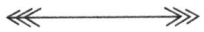

THE NEXT MORNING, I learned that the best time for a motorhome to break is in the fall when the peak travel season is coming to a close and thousands of vehicles are being tucked away for the winter. By the time ours busted for the third time, it was high time in camper season, midway through May.

"Yeah. Uh..." There was a long pause on the phone. Some typing. "I could fit you in maybe next week if we wrap up a diesel we're working on, but definitely in two weeks. How's Thursday, May 27 for you?"

The twenty-seventh was fifteen days away. How far along the route would I even be at that point? "Yeah, I can't do that. I'm running across America for my mom. Can you recommend any other shops?"

"I mean, it's all going to be the same," the man on the phone said. "There's four other shops in town, but there's a good chance they're all booked too. This is just how it is this time of year."

I sighed, digging my finger into the crease of my nail bed.

"Listen," he said, "I know a guy who does stuff on the side. His name is Stew. It won't be certified, but he may be able to take a look."

I wrote down his number.

The night before, after Nate had called from the side of I-80, the three of us stood in the dark in forty-degree rain while a tow truck big enough to pull a semi arrived. It reversed into position, beeping as big trucks do, and hoisted the front of our rig onto a platform before the driver chained it into place. I had him tow it to an RV resort in Park City, the direction we were headed, so we had a place to sleep that night, and so I could also keep running along the route the next morning. Shortly after 9:00 a.m., I called the first shop listed on Google, hoping for a lucky break. Stew's number was that break, but it would cost us. The radiator was leaking, and he had to take the engine apart to fix it. And now, again, the generator didn't work.

For the third time in less than two months, I called the family that owned the vehicle with news about more repairs.

"Hi, Mary Ann!" I said, trying to sound chipper but not too cheerful.

"Ashley," she replied through the phone, "how are you? How's the run?"

The little time I knew of Mary Ann and her family made these conversations difficult for me. I felt like all I did was call them to ask for help and money to fix their camper. My unease had less to do with them—they were always more than gracious—and more to do with my need to move through life independently.

Mary Ann was the sister of the man who owned the vehicle—a guy named Joe who lived in Chicago. Their cousin had MS, and Joe hadn't used the motorhome in years because of health problems of his own. It sat on their land in Wild Rose, Wisconsin, where my aunt lived until she hosted a polka pancake breakfast and So-and-So who knew So-and-So said there was a motorhome parked on their land. The rest was history, though it hadn't gone as smoothly as I had hoped.

After a quick tune-up of the vehicle and rundown of how to operate it, Nate and I had it for only a matter of days, driving it out to the start, before it needed thousands of dollars of work in Utah for shocks and tires. Then I busted the spare tire hitch in Tahoe. And now it was the radiator. My guess was they had put more into it than it was worth, but somehow, that didn't seem to matter.

"Oh gosh, that thing's got you stuck again," Mary Ann said. "What a pain. Don't worry about a thing, Ashley. Let me get my credit card." I could hear her rustling around in her purse.

"Mary Ann. I just… I don't know what to say," I said through the phone. A knot tightened in my stomach.

"Oh, it's just money," she replied. "It comes and goes. I want to take my grandbabies out in that thing when you get back, and you're doing me a huge favor by working out all the kinks."

I was hardly doing her any favors, I knew, but I didn't argue. I took her card number, then thanked God for her and her family. It pained me to admit it, but I needed their support. I had eleven more states to run.

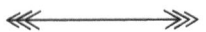

THE THREE DAYS IT took Stew to repair the motorhome can only be described as prickly. It didn't take long before I had run as far as I could from Park City before it was too far to drive back and forth between the route and where our camper sat, so we sat too. I wasn't logging miles, the repairs were timely and expensive, and Nate's frustration with the endeavor—its monotony and inconveniences—only continued to mount.

Sitting in a coffee shop with both Nate and Spade on the third morning adrift, it got worse.

"Hi, this is Lydia from B&H Photography calling," the woman said to me through the phone. "I just need to verify the shipping address of your credit card before sending out your order."

At a table with the guys, I stood to take the call outside, away from the bustling espresso machine.

"I'm sorry," I replied, standing alone on the sidewalk, staring at a snowy range of mountain peaks. "Can you tell me the order first?"

My pulse quickened.

"Sure! Let's see, we have an SLR lens for $679 and a mirrorless digital for $649. The total is $1,328, plus shipping and tax."

I looked back at Spade through the window, the only photographer I knew who had my nonprofit's credit card number. It was the one I reluctantly gave him back in Sacramento when he asked to borrow money for his flight to Alaska.

"I've got the ticket pulled up on the computer," he had said. "Want to just rattle off the numbers, and I'll get it booked?"

I hesitated but then read him the numbers out loud. The ease with which he suggested it made me feel guilty for even thinking I shouldn't. He was volunteering for my event, taking professional pictures for free, sleeping on a motorhome couch. Did I not trust him?

He sat next to Nate now, typing on his laptop, unfazed by my departure.

"Cancel the order," I said to the lady on the phone. "I never placed it. It's fraud."

Pulling the coffeehouse door open to return inside, I had no plan. It was just *Get to the table. Confront Spade. Try not to explode.*

"What's up, babe? Who was that?" Nate asked, reading my face.

"That was a woman from B&H Photography," I said, staring at Spade. "Verifying my shipping address for an order."

Spade looked up from his screen. His eyebrows furrowed. "Why would they be calling you?"

"I don't know, Spade. Maybe because the credit card is in my name. Why are you using the credit card number I gave you to buy equipment?"

"What? Oh God," he said, throwing up his empty palms as if I had a gun, "I'm not. I don't even make purchases. My accountant handles all my transactions."

"Well, how did your accountant get the number?" I pressed.

"I don't know. He keeps all the information since I'm on the road so much. He must have mixed up the numbers. I'll call him right away," he said, pulling out his phone, pressing buttons, then putting it to his ear. "Check the account. Have there been any other transactions?"

I, too, had an accountant. An hour later, I received an Excel spreadsheet bright with yellow boxes. He'd highlighted all the transactions that didn't fit my route—a mess of purchases ranging from dinners in Alaska to equipment in California. A total of $5,277.

"I don't care what it takes," I said sternly to Spade, still at the coffee shop but ready to leave. "I want every last dollar returned to the nonprofit. Now."

I closed my laptop and stood, pushing the chair back across the floor. Its wooden legs screeched across the tile. What was I even doing? Clearly, I couldn't manage a nonprofit, a business where people willfully gave someone their money so it could be put to good, charitable use.

And I was trying to raise how much? Five hundred thousand dollars? Really? I couldn't even manage the $16,439 I happened to bring in so far, a third of which was now tied up in fraudulent purchases. People who were successful didn't lose $5,277 and not notice. People who knew what the fuck they were doing looked at the numbers.

I didn't do that. I ran. I was a runner. I didn't even consider having an accountant until someone introduced me to one.

"You should really have a CPA reconcile the monthly funds," an acquaintance had suggested.

I replied foolishly, "What's reconciling the funds mean?"

The man paused, considering how to explain it to a twenty-five-year-old who had had no accounting or business experience. "It means someone would make sure that the funds that come in match up with the expenses that go out."

I nodded, not knowing why we would need that, not thinking of where else funds would go. Later, I would have to Google the term "CPA."

Now, I was thankful for my volunteer CPA, knowing exactly where funds could go with me giving the credit card to a nomadic photographer.

We will reconcile Spade's purchases, I thought, trying out the sophisticated term in my mind. They were found, after all, aglow on the spreadsheet, hidden among the thousands of dollars I recently donated—the $8,000 check for research, among others. I expected large sums of money to be gone from the account, but still. If the woman from B&H hadn't called, who knows how much would have been taken?

Following me outside, Spade apologized again. "Ashley, I'm so sorry about this mix-up." He said, "It's such a mess. I'll get it all straightened out. Okay?"

"I know you will," I said, looking at him. Challenging him to tell me anything different.

"Listen, I know it's the money you're trying to raise," he said. "Give me a few days. Okay? I know how important this is for you. For your family."

At the mention of my family, I softened. He'd met my mother. He knew exactly what this was all about. He watched us walk her, hands under her arms for support, on the uneven ground of my parents' backyard for family photos. Did traveling photographers have their accountants make their purchases? I didn't know. Why did he come back if he stole it on purpose? Surely this was all a mistake.

"Okay. It's just... I should have noticed sooner, that's all. I'm mad at myself. But we need that money back."

Leaving the coffee shop, the three of us drove straight to Salt Lake City to pick up the motorhome, which was now fixed, then moved the caravan forward to Strawberry Adventures RV Park along Highway 40—a remote campground tucked beneath plateaus of layered red earth, 86.5 miles away from the city.

"We can't trust him," Nate whispered to me while I helped him outside, hooking up the water hose. He unlocked the side compartment, lifting the panel door open. "I knew something was off ever since he came to Wisconsin, sleeping all morning in the basement. Who does that?"

"He said he can get us the money back," I whispered in return, watching around the back corner of the RV while Nate pulled out the water connection. "If he was trying to steal money, why did he come back?"

Nate shook his head. "I don't know. I just have a feeling."

Nate's feelings, though, were something I couldn't count on lately. After fifty-three days on the road, they were all over the map. Having met Anne and Gundy and experiencing their seamless setup, a floodgate opened in his mind.

"We need to get a tow hitch like they have," Nate had said the day after they passed us on the highway. "It'll save so much time on the days we move. Right now, it's a huge waste of time—driving you to run, driving back, getting the motorhome, driving forward, then setting up camp all over again. With a hitch, we just link up and go forward."

"We're not getting a tow hitch. Those things are like $3,500."

"Can't you ask Montel?" he said.

"Nate, his sponsor is paying for gas, our food, all of this," I said, sweeping my hand in the air while we sat inside the RV. "What more do you want?"

"I want a tow hitch so I don't have to drive for an extra two hours every three days."

"Who cares about two hours of driving? Do you have somewhere else to be?" I asked.

He clenched his jaw, then stood to go outside, pushing the motorhome door closed with *umph*.

I couldn't figure out what his problem was—he was now irritated about the "extra" miles, angry at the mechanical issues, bored by the redundancy of our days. He had a surprising, unexpected need to move along, and all I could think was *To where?*

I needed to talk with someone more stable. I needed my father.

"Dad, what should I do?" I asked over the phone. I took the call on a walk away from our campsite, near a trickling creek. Under different circumstances, I'd have been quite blissful here—standing on a patch of bright grass, a stream of water nearby, colored rocky earth towering above me. We were on the cusp of summer, and I could smell freshness in the air.

"Right now, you do nothing," he said. "You play nice. The best thing you can hope for is to get that money back, and you can't do that if Spade gets mad and takes off."

Thankfully, everything had happened at a time when we could keep an eye on Spade. It wouldn't be impossible if he wanted to leave—sneaking out in the middle of the night from the couch that was directly across from the door, heading to the highway that was just feet from our campsite to hitchhike or hoof it to the city. But it was certainly more difficult now that we had moved the caravan out of the city and I had asked him to keep his luggage in the trunk of the locked car to free up space in the motorhome.

I returned to the campsite, where Nate sat at the picnic table with Spade. "All right, what can I make for dinner?" I asked cheerfully as if nothing was amiss.

As long as the money was returned, all would be well.

CHAPTER ELEVEN
Settled Dust

THE NEXT MORNING, SPADE was on the couch. He didn't sneak off into the night; he stayed right where I had last seen him. He smiled at me when I came out of the bathroom and offered to make me coffee.

"Ah, I'll pass," I said. "I still haven't crossed over to the dark side."

He laughed. "Fair enough. I'll boil the water for your tea."

The weather outside had shifted back to spring, the sky being an overcast of gray clouds that flecked tiny sprinkles of water across the window. Early May in the north always seemed to be a tug-of-war between fleeting spring and advancing summer.

And I, of course, was anxious to run. My heel bobbed up and down under the dinette table like a piston while I ate my creamy peanut-butter-and-craisin oatmeal. It had been three days since I had last run, and I was looking forward to making up some miles and easing the flurry of thoughts that whipped around my mind.

"Do you think it would be okay if I stayed here?" Spade asked as I tied my shoe by the couch. "I've got a few calls to make, and my reception was spotty in the canyons. I want to make sure the funds are transferred today."

I looked up at Nate, who was sitting in the chair across from me. Since we found out the money had been missing, we hadn't let Spade out of our sight.

"You can stay here if you let us take your camera equipment and driver's license," Nate said.

I tilted my head. "Is that necessary?" I asked Nate, playing the good guy, though I would have never thought of that brilliant solution myself. Nate was street-smart, and I wanted Spade to think I believed everything he told me.

"Hey, look, man," Nate said to Spade, "I'm happy to believe this was all a mistake once the money is returned. But until then, it'd be silly of me to think otherwise."

"That's fair, man," Spade said in return. "It's cool. You can take my stuff."

Out on the road with Nate, while Spade stayed back, I eased into the run. Highway 40 was the main line between Salt Lake City and the towns directly east of it—Heber City, Duchense, and Vernal—as well as the smaller, unincorporated ones in between.

The shoulder I ran along was neither cramped nor generous. It was a paved space half a car's width with a flat patch of dirt on its border, and I was grateful for it.

Running against traffic in my neon-yellow reflective vest, I carefully watched the drivers coming at me, though I could do nothing for those at my back. The first time a car from behind passed another car going the same direction, I felt a whoosh of steel speed past my body so unexpectedly that I jumped into the ditch out of fright. The eighteen-wheelers never did that, generally being more careful of pedestrian traffic, but cars weren't so careful, or worse, weren't paying attention, and both were the type that could get me killed. I ran without music because I enjoyed myself just the same without it, but part of me wondered: *If this was how I go, would it help if I didn't hear it?*

The landscape stole my attention from such lingering thoughts. The reddened rocky earth at the campground continued, colored by hardy green shrubs and patches of periwinkle flower blooms. I ran at 5,700-feet elevation on a steady incline, on my way to Duchense at 6,600, and every so often, that incline was guarded by a steel rail. On the other side, I'd find a gully or land that led to a gully—an erosion of rusted earth that appeared like a valley formed by torrential water. The steel rail ran along the same line that I ran, pushing me onto the road until a car or semi appeared up ahead. When this happened and there was land on the other side of the guard, I'd hurdle the railing and walk along the tightrope space between the gully and the rail until the vehicle passed. When there was a gully and no land, I'd sprint until the railing met the land, then I'd jump.

I ran, and I watched. I ran, and I listened. I ran, and I hurdled, feeling grateful to be distracted. Every three miles, I came upon the car.

"Spade did it on purpose," Nate said with conviction, cantering toward me. The Camry was pulled over on the westbound side of the road in a grassy gravel clearing.

"What? Why would you say that?" I asked, catching my breath.

"I found this," he said, handing me a thin receipt. "It's a credit card receipt from one of Spade's transactions in Alaska. I had to wait until the place was open, but I just called them. They remember him."

"You did?" I asked, "What'd they say?"

A semi passed, gushing us with its tailwind. The receipt fluttered in my fingertips.

"The manager got the waitress who ran the transaction," he explained. "She described him perfectly—his hat, his hair color, his goatee. She said he told her he lost his credit card the day before on a remote photo shoot, but he had the number memorized and wrote it down on a piece of paper. The card wasn't declined, so she figured his story was true."

I said nothing, standing there, stunned.

I couldn't fathom it—that Spade flew to Wisconsin to photograph my family, that he met my mother, that he stared down his lens into her kind, gentle eyes, then stole money from the charity founded to help people like her and had the nerve to lie to my face about it. Who would do that?

"B-b-but why did he come back?" I stammered. There was so much of me that *still* didn't want to believe it was true.

"I don't know, but he made a huge mistake doing so," Nate said. "I want to go back to the campground and beat the shit out of him."

"Fuck," I whispered with a sigh. "We can't. Nate, we need that money back. What do we do? Call the cops?"

"I don't know. What are the cops going to do?"

"Fuck." I was dumbfounded into speaking only swear words. "I've gotta call my dad."

Sitting in the car with Nate, I dialed his number.

"Dad," I said, my voice shaking, tears brimming in my eyes, "I'm so mad right now. What do I do?" I had spit out the story in one long sentence, hardly stopping for a breath.

He spoke evenly. He knew exactly what to say. "Take a few deep breaths and act normal. See if he's good for the money. Hopefully, he is. That's the best you can go for. Then, drop him off on the side of the road and don't look back."

"Should I call the cops? He stole from us, Dad. That's illegal." I sounded like the child that I was.

"Meister," he replied, using his pet name for me, knowing who I was and what I preferred to do—that I was seeing red and was ready for revenge. "You can't take this on. Do you plan on fighting him in court while you run across the country? You don't need that. Just kick him to the curb and forget about it."

"He could do this to someone else?" My voice rose. "We have to stop it."

"Ashley, you can't take on the world," he said. "One thing at a time. What you're doing now is plenty enough. You've got to focus on what you're out there for."

While he spoke, I opened the car door and started to pace back and forth on the grassy gravel patch. The sky began to drizzle again. If anyone knew how to reason with me, it was my father, though even that took patience. I was seven when my brother swore at my mother and she washed his mouth out with soap. At the time, my brother was my best friend, so to teach her a lesson, I vowed to scream as loud as I could until she apologized. She took me to my room, screaming until, an hour later, I fell asleep from exhaustion. When I awoke, I didn't talk to her for a week. For better or worse, I had a convicted heart. It was difficult to sway.

Just then, my phone vibrated with an incoming call. It was

Spade. "Dad, I gotta go. He's calling. Call you back."
I switched the line.
"Hey, man," I said, trying to make my shaking voice sound cheerful, "what's going on?"
"Hey! A transfer of $4,000 just went through. It should be in your account. I can do the remaining $2,000 in a day or so. I tagged on a little extra on for all the trouble," he said.
"Great." I nodded yes to Nate, gesturing good news. "Just finishing up out here for the morning. We'll see you shortly."

That the money was in the account gave me hope. Hope that I wasn't a complete idiot. Hope that I could get the full sum back, and in doing so, it would lessen the severity of what was actually happening–which was that I had met a criminal in an airport and simply trusted him to be exactly who he said he was, as I had trusted everyone else.

What he had done was beyond me, being someone who had a hard time even lying to get an entry-level cashier job in college. My friend had been smart, falsifying her availability so she could earn cash before spring break. The thought of lying about my availability never even crossed my mind.

She started earning money, and I kept looking for work, frustrated with myself for not being clever enough to have done the same.

Sitting in the car on the way back to the campground, I stared out the window in a daze. I had been foolish. Nate did a wise thing, finding evidence to back up Spade's story while I laced up my shoes to run, itching to feel better. Even in our cruise ship roles, I was cocooned in a happy place where children and families came to play. Sure, people went to the casino to play too, but at the casino, there was money, and where there was money, there was greed. No one came to the rock wall to pull one over on me. My biggest concern had been keeping people safe.

In his years as a dealer at the casino, Nate had learned to be both friendly and watchful, spending hours looking for subtle inconsistencies. He had used this sense with Spade, feeling something was off and trusting it. And I brushed him aside, choosing rather to believe that this volunteer photographer was a godsend, as all the others had been on this destined journey for charity.

I thought about Spade's quick reaction in the coffee shop, wondering how he came up with an explanation so quickly, and then mulling over how hurried I was to believe him. Nobody wants to be taken advantage of. Believing that I hadn't been was simply more tolerable than considering otherwise.

Spade wasn't a godsend. Nate was. This adventure hadn't been as seamless as I had dreamed it up to him, but here he was protecting me all the same. I grabbed his hand as we rode along, and he squeezed mine back, giving me a warm, half smile.

We'll be okay, his eyes said.

And I knew, with him at my side, that was something I could believe.

Back at the campground, I took a long, hot shower, making sure to empty the gray holding tank so that it wouldn't back up. I didn't cycle the water, turning off the spray while I soaped as I had been regularly doing. Instead, I stood underneath the water and let the heat beat at my shoulders. I needed to be alone for a moment, to stand under the water and breathe. To let the heat rush over my face and wash the day away.

I took a deep breath in and blew out. If you had asked me what running across America would be like, this was not it.

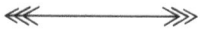

"**WHAT ELSE WILL I** have to do except run?" I said to a reporter questioning my thoughts about the endeavor. She was a marathon runner herself and knew what twenty to thirty miles a day for six months might feel like.

"I'll have the whole day to run, eat, and rest," I told her. "There will be plenty of time to recover."

When I quit my job on the cruise ship and came home to do this, that's what I imagined—that there'd be running and plenty of time. Yes, I'd be running a long way, but still just running, and that alone would raise half a million dollars. People would hear about my mother's story and my effort to make an impact, and they'd give. The money would simply come in.

Founding the nonprofit happened out of convenience because the sponsors who would line up for the event would want tax exemption, and no charities were willing to partner with me in that way. I would start my own, simply, and at that, the problem was solved. But a nonprofit is not simply a platform to receive tax exemption for a donation. It's a business. There are quarterly tax returns, donor receipts, bylaws, and rules. Had I known exactly what it was, maybe I would have given it some thought. Had I known that I wouldn't be just running, maybe I would have been better prepared.

Shortly after I finished building the organization's website and hit Publish, I started pacing back and forth in my childhood bedroom, sweating. How many people would submit questions through the contact form? Would I have enough time to answer all the inquiries and also train? The next day, when I woke up, there were not hundreds of hits on the site. There was one, and it was my own. That was the moment that I realized hundreds of people were not feverishly searching "running across America" as I had been. I chuckled at myself, slightly relieved that I didn't have to reply to hundreds of messages, and went for a run.

The messages did come, though. Not while I trained as I had anticipated, but now, while I ran across the country. It wasn't just running. It was running, managing vehicle repairs, finding a place to park, replying to emails and social media messages, writing blog posts, and scheduling interviews with the media. The month before I left was a frenzy, and in addition to receiving the motorhome and sponsorship support, Fox Sports Wisconsin wanted to air weekly updates of my run during MLB Brewers games. A three-minute update of my progress would be viewed by over one hundred thousand people every week for six months. I got butterflies just thinking about it before the start. Not for the notoriety but for the donations.

Maybe I should increase my fundraising goal, I thought.

How silly.

I checked the account. The $4,000 that Spade transferred was there, much to my relief, alongside the measly $17,647 in donations that had been given so far. If I were going to raise half a million dollars by my finish in New York, I'd better get to it.

I let the hot water massage my muscles. There was so much to do, and now this. Spade stole from the charity and was lying about it. The fact that he was here was both a gift and a bit weird. We actually had a chance at being refunded, but I felt like a fake myself—carrying on friendly conversation, laughing at his stupid fucking jokes, picking up his lunch plate, and washing it in the sink to appear as if nothing were amiss while knowing who he really was. Doing it made my skin crawl, like walking across a thin sheet of ice upon a deep lake.

The best possible result depended on my will to move cautiously—*slowly*—with light ease across an unstable plane. I couldn't make a break for it as I wanted to. I could make no sudden movements. The crackling of breaking ground spoke to me the truth of where I stood. I could only do as I had been doing, inching forward, acting as if the entire surface would not drop beneath me and swallow me whole.

I squeezed a glob of rosemary mint shampoo into my palm and rubbed my hands together, then lathered it into my hair. The smell settled me, transporting me to someplace refreshing. I first learned to do this when I arrived back at my parents' home and saw that the bathroom wasn't spared from the plethora of things my father hoarded or left unfixed. The medicine cabinet above the sink was no longer mirrored as it had once been; rather, it was a large oak box with four shelves that had hinges for a mirror that was now gone. Its shelves weren't so much a space for a variety of medicines but rather for a line of twelve empty deodorant sticks my father was saving to scrape the remains from and collect together in one stick so as not to be wasteful. Their caps collected dust.

He had these complexities of collecting, and that confused and irritated me, but these feelings were eased by all the other ways in which he was absolutely divine. He was a man of deep character, one who showed up in every other way that didn't require him to be tidy. For my mother, it was doing things like changing her from her evening Depends every morning into a pair of underwear for the day, then helping her over and over again to the bathroom on the days she couldn't fully do it herself.

SETTLED DUST

Certainly, it would have been easier just to keep her in Depends throughout the day, but he cared not only about her but also about her dignity. I saw this in a hundred ways he tended her, then a hundred more—the way he dyed her hair every six weeks because she couldn't herself, that he topped the bird feeders every morning and fed the feral neighborhood cat in the afternoon because she asked him to, that he'd bring her along each and every time he left the house, even when it was much easier not to.

In recent times, it was to coast along in the car while I trained for the endeavor, just to watch me run. For my mother, it was an adventure away from the couch, and for my father, the mowing could wait. I'd smile and wave. They'd smile and wave back. This doting skewed my reality to believe that those who loved me would be happy just to watch.

The day that I ran my first fifty-mile race, I tiptoed down the stairs after my alarm went off at 3:00 a.m. to find them standing in the kitchen with steaming coffee in their to-go mugs.

"You ready, kid?" my father said. His hair was brushed damp against his head. He had already showered.

In the car, surrounded by darkness while we drove to the race start, I sat in the backseat staring at my mother's face illuminated by the dull blue light cast from the dashboard, wondering about her days. It had been a decade since she could drive or go anywhere on her own. The depth of her independence was that she could still move about the house on "good days" with her hand along the wall, for which we were grateful. She awoke in the wee hours of the morning to see me run, or was it something else? Looking at the outline of her content face, I had no doubt she'd wake up at any time, day or night, just for a chance to get out of the house.

Running the race, I saw them at every point of entry to the trail. Nine miles after the start at the first aid station, we all had a good chuckle when I pulled soaking wet socks from my drop bag—it had rained, and I hadn't known yet to place my supplies in plastic bags.

I ran off into the woods, unfazed by the socks, and they took off as well, driving to the nearest town to buy me new ones, doing anything they could to help me finish. I saw them at the road crossings, my father clapping and my mother waving overenthusiastically from the open car window. At mile thirty, my father walked at my side for a short stretch.

"All right," I said, tucking a half-eaten granola bar into my water bottle pocket. "Let's see how this goes. I've never run this far before. Twenty miles left."

"I felt strong about the distance I had covered and also apprehensive of the ones ahead. How would I feel? How bad would it hurt? How would I manage myself if the pain became too much?

"It's not twenty miles, Meister. It's just one," my father said, patting me once firmly on the back. "Run one mile at a time, and I'll see you at the finish."

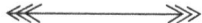

I RINSED THE ROSEMARY mint shampoo from my hair and reached for the conditioner. I took another deep breath and felt better.

I would no longer think about what was lost if Spade took off or, worse, if he stayed and tried to hurt us. I wouldn't think about how I'd possibly raise half a million dollars or the thousands who were watching me try. I wouldn't think about how Nate and I would manage the vehicles, my running, his frustrations, and a nonprofit business alone for the next four months.

I would only think of the very next thing.

I'd finish my hair and wash my body. I'd towel myself off and cover my skin in cocoa butter lotion. I'd get dressed and brush my teeth. And then I'd step into the thirty-foot-by-eight-foot box I shared with a thief and wait him out. As my father had taught me to, as he had done so himself, the best of me arrived when I focused on the mile I was in.

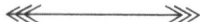

LATER THAT AFTERNOON, CLEANED and rested, I received a new message through the website's contact form. It wasn't the hundreds

I had imagined would come in, but not a day went by when someone didn't contact me to thank me, encourage me, or offer to meet me along the route. That's how I met the Rouskas, though the story of how Jen came across my information was certainly interesting.

"Okay, don't think this is weird." She laughed loudly, standing in a semicircle with her husband, Nate, Spade, and me on the side of the highway. "But on our third day of driving back and forth to a hockey tournament in Salt Lake City and seeing you run along Highway 40, I made Bryan pull the car over at the campground at like midnight so I could sneak up and write down your website."

The fact that she was creeping around the camper at midnight and I hadn't known was mildly unnerving, given that a thief was also sleeping on my couch. But she was Jen, and Jen was a smiley, spunky platinum-blond woman with a pixie cut mohawk. She bounced out of her truck toward me after coaxing her husband and two children to drive out and meet us the day after we found out about Spade's deceit. As residents of Vernal, the next town along my route, Jen sent me an email asking if she could join me for a run.

Why not? I thought. I figured that Spade would stay at the RV again, and I could enjoy ten miles with a fellow runner. Except Spade didn't stay at the RV. He offered to come along and take pictures, and now that the miles with her were complete, we all stood together talking. I tried to wrap up the conversation now with a transition into needing to eat.

"Oh! Well, you have to come for dinner," she said. "My parents might swing by, and we can't ever tell them how we met because we're Mormon, and they'd flip if they knew I met you on the internet, but you have to come for dinner."

Spade stood to my left. I changed the subject. "You're Mormon? Do they allow mohawks?"

She laughed a boisterous roar, running her hand through her purple-highlighted hair. "Ah, yeah. I'm a little wild for them, but they still let me in church." I realized then I had no idea what being Mormon meant. My only references were the pairs of suited men I saw occasionally knocking at my parents' door and a kid in my elementary school whose mother was Mormon, neither of which looked anything like Jen.

"Okay, but really," she said, "you have to come for dinner. You can park the RV out front, and I'll do your laundry."

A knot formed in my stomach. "I don't know," I said. "It's not that I don't want to. It's just I really like to get the RV hooked up before dark. We do pretty early mornings." I hated lying to her. I wanted nothing more than to go to her house. To have her do my laundry. For her to make us dinner.

"Well, don't hook the RV up. You can stay at our place," she said. "Right, Bryan? You don't mind if they stay, do you?"

"Yeah, you should stay," he said.

What a great pair—her spunky and fun, him charming and friendly. Their two early teen children stood at their side, looking mildly interested at the woman their mother found on the internet.

"We have a guest room, and we'll make Maddie stay in Cade's room. He has bunks. They'll love it, right, guys?" he said to the kids.

Cade shrugged his shoulders, indifferent, as teenage boys are. "Sure."

"That sounds great," Spade said before I could come up with a reason not to. "We should stay." He looked at me.

Fuck.

An hour later, my throat tightened as I watched Spade photograph the kids jumping on the giant backyard trampoline. We pulled up at the address Jen texted me and parked the RV in front of a massive home in a new development. Their three-car garage was big enough for their truck, their SUV, and the pair of four-wheelers they used on the trails. A rack with four mountain bikes hung from the side wall. Dried red dirt covered the tire treads. I imagined them taking the bikes off the wall, buckling their helmets on, and riding in a line of four up and over the hills. Once again, it was everything I ever wanted for my family—the home, the mobility, the hours of recreation together. The bitterness I felt toward what wasn't ours was, at times, palpable. With it, there'd always be fuel to run.

Bryan flipped the chicken on their gas grill with a pair of tongs on the patio of their sprawling suburban home while the kids bounced. Nate stood at his side, enjoying a beer. Jen made a salad in the kitchen. Spade's shutter clicked.

"Hey, you want to help me get the laundry?" I said to Nate. "I think there's a few loads. We should get those started."

He looked at me, and I nodded to the side. He nodded back, knowing we should talk.

Once inside the motorhome, feeling sneaky and like someone might somehow overhear us, I lowered my voice. "We need to eat and leave. We have to get Spade out of their home."

He nodded in agreement, feeling the tension.

"What do we do?" he whispered back. "Do you think we can say something like it's easier to run in the morning if we have the camper set up? Something about getting out really early and not wanting to wake them?"

"I don't know. Jen's pretty persistent. Do you think I should just tell her what's going on?"

Nate shook his head slowly. "I don't know, babe. What are they going to think of us?"

I pushed the nail from one hand into the nail bed of my thumb. A shot of pain ran along the side of my finger, and it dulled the growing anxiety. It was a fidgety habit I'd picked up years ago, standing at the starting line of cross-country meets, coursing with adrenaline.

"I think we've got to tell them," I said in reply, feeling it to be the right thing to do. "Even if they hate us for bringing him here, at least they'll know and can come up with some reason to ask us to leave without him thinking anything of it."

He agreed. We gathered the dirty laundry and went inside.

When it came to it, the only advice of my father that I didn't follow was when he told me not to look back after dropping Spade on the side of the road—that, I did.

After dinner, when I went on a walk with Jen to tell her, she and Bryan insisted that we stay so they could help. After the remaining funds were returned to the bank account the next morning, the four of us stood before Spade and told him what we knew. After we threw his things in the car, drove him to the far edge of town, and dropped him at a bus stop, it was then that I looked back to watch the dust kick up from the car on him standing there, bag in the dirt, with his paperboy cap in his hand.

That's what the wolf looks like, I willed myself to remember as I watched him shrink. *They dress in sheep's clothing.*

CHAPTER TWELVE

Colorful Colorado

THE HARPSICHORD'S GENTLE METALLIC vibrations sounded from my phone. I reached over in the darkness of the morning and hit snooze, then settled back into my pillow. I fell back into the comfort of a nothingness sleep, where the reality of the past week didn't exist, where nothing did. When I slept, I slept hard—completely gone from the world. On the morning of May 20, eight weeks into my run across the country, being gone from the reality of this event was exactly what I wanted.

An hour or so later (I didn't know), my eyes opened to the day's brightness shining through the motorhome's closed window shade. The sun appeared like an upbeat friend with a sympathy plant, and I sighed.

With Spade gone, the Rouskas had invited us to stay as long as we wanted to, and we did, until the miles that I ran stretched so far from their home, through town and across another state line, that we could no longer avoid our departure. We had moved on from the Rouskas' comfort. And comfortable it was.

They had fed us, washed our laundry, and cleaned our caravan as a family—soaping up a sponge and chasing each other around the driveway with it, laughing all the while.

When I showered, I couldn't touch the ceiling. When I brushed my teeth, my forehead didn't knock the mirror. When I flushed the toilet, my waste disappeared, never to be tended to by me again. These conveniences came with an ease of being cared for that both Nate and I enjoyed, along with what seemed to be his deepest yearning that our setup didn't fulfill–sports on cable TV. He had lain across their plush leather couch for the last time in front of a sixty-four-inch flat screen watching tennis, then we packed our things and dragged on.

Nate rolled over and draped his arm across my stomach. "Thanks for the extra sleep, babe," he said. "It feels good to rest."

He didn't know. I wasn't resting. I was hiding.

Spade was gone, but everything that had happened from his being here remained. If it weren't for Nate, he'd still be sleeping on the couch, stealing from my nonprofit. How stupid was I? I wasn't inspiring. I was naive. He probably picked me out at that airport—me skipping around the terminal with a dumb smile on my face for being on national television. I had replayed our meeting over and over in my mind. The way he started up the conversation, the way I offered information.

We sat at a table near the gates, looking over his photos. He talked, and I nodded, staring at the glossy prints. The sun setting perfectly on the cowgirl while her horse skidded around a barrel, kicking up sand. Her gun stretched out from a steady hand.

He could do that for my run, I thought. I saw what I wanted to.

Welcome to Colorful Colorado said a massive wooden sign the day before, when we pulled into Dinosaur, Colorado, after leaving Jen and Bryan's. We set up camp at Blue Mountain Village RV Park. I felt many things, but colorful was not one of them.

Parking the RV in its spot, I was at least grateful for the electrical and water hookups. Without them, we'd run electricity off the generator, an engine below the couch that sounded like a tractor, which is what I thought we'd have to do when we pulled our vehicles into the worn town of Dinosaur.

Of the RV park's name, I couldn't see anything that resembled blue mountains or a park. We shared a dust-covered pad next to a few permanent trailers and an impressive anthill. As we set up, I glanced at it, watching the ants walk up and down, up and down, in a straight line carrying tiny white balls.

I glanced across the stretch of land toward the south. It was a field of similar mounds. Just before sundown, a motorcycle rally rode in. Their group of fifty-some riders set up camp too, then played classic rock music, and drank until who knows a.m.

Now the morning had come, as it does, unfazed by my sulking. The miles pulled me out of bed the way I imagine a young child would at times with their parent, tugging at me.

Some days are a slog to life.

I mixed a spoonful of creamy peanut butter into my oatmeal with a pour of hot water. The metal spoon scraped the side of the ceramic bowl and delivered to my mouth the same glob that I'd eaten every morning since the coast. Nate emerged, finally, from the bathroom, and I stood from the dinette to take his place.

"Sorry," he said. "You might want to give it a few minutes. My stomach couldn't wait."

"I can't," I said, turning sideways to pass him in the narrow hall. I'd hold my breath.

And I did.

After wiping with stiff, one-ply toilet paper, a suggested product for the RV's holding tanks, I stepped on the lever that opened the bowl to the shit water just below. I grabbed my toothbrush and left the space.

The paste foamed in my mouth, and I spit it into the empty kitchen sink, using the faucet to wash it down.

"Could you not do that over the clean dishes?" Nate asked.

"I'm not. The dishes are over there," I replied, pointing to the other side of the sink—the one we used as a drying space. I rinsed my toothbrush and returned it to the bathroom.

The day looked more summer than spring, so I dressed in a royal-blue sweat-wicking T-shirt and dark shorts. I reached for an airy running jacket that hung in the closet, just in case, and then walked to the couch to put on my socks.

"You know we're going to need a tow for the car now, right?" Nate said.

I fiddled with my socks, wanting to avoid the subject. "I'll poke around," I replied. I still didn't see the need, but I had little motivation to debate it and even less ammo, except that it cost more than what I wanted to pay (which was nothing).

The topic had been pushed back since Nevada. When he'd bring it up, I'd tell him how much easier it would be once Spade returned. We'd have an extra driver to move vehicles and a helping hand to crew. He'd even be able to sleep in a few times a week, I told him.

And now, well.

I set my shoes by the door and stuffed the peanut-butter-and-jelly sandwich I made in a plastic sandwich bag, ready to run.

In the car, just before 10:00 a.m., we drove out of the sleepy Blue Mountain Village RV Park onto a road called Stegosaurus Freeway. A tattered single-story home with a tin roof sat on its corner, and I looked at it out of the passenger side window while Nate took the driver's seat. Its lawn was a spattering of patchy, browned grass. The car's blinker tick-clicked while we waited for a Ford F-150 to pass.

Into town a few blocks later, we passed a stegosaurus statue on the left and Christie's Liquor on the right, then headed west on Highway 40 toward Vernal. We drove by a cluster of new sheds for sale and a large highway pullout until we arrived at a smaller highway pullout. The exact place I finished the day before, just a mile or so out of town.

"Okay," Nate said, coming to a stop. He shifted the center stick into park.

Opening the door, I propped my foot on the frame to tie the laces of my Asics, then grabbed the water bottle that was in the center console, mixed with the only drink powder the product sponsor had sent me—fruit punch, again.

"I'll find a spot a couple miles up the road," he said once I had gathered my gear.

"Sounds good. Thanks." I closed the door and stood in a world of crispy sagebrush and hard sand. The car pulled away.

Walking at first, I squinted at the sun overhead. It was late morning and hot. No longer were there signs of a lingering spring day. I wouldn't need the airy jacket I placed in the back seat after all. I wore sunglasses, but the height of the sun peeked brightness in through the top. I pushed the glasses further up my nose, and my eyelashes brushed the lens. The color of the earth had changed suddenly—from the reddened chunks of rock gathered in plateaus in Utah to a dried, bland crust blotted with sprouts of parched, sad grass. Everything seemed to be just a bit scorched.

Attempting to lift my mood before starting to run, I pulled out my phone and posted on Facebook. After all, I had run to my beloved Colorado.

How cool, I reminded myself.

"I've run to Colorado. My life is complete," I typed, though I certainly didn't feel complete. Those who read the post would never know about Spade, and neither would those following the blog. After some consideration, I'd decided not to mention it. There were too many people following the event, too many stories emerging about kind people giving generously—Montel and the sponsorship, Joe donating the RV and its repairs, the Turners with the car, people like Jen and Bryan opening their home. I saw how these acts of giving restored a sense of goodness in people that made my mother proud. I didn't want one bad seed to spoil the bunch.

"See?" I could imagine some people saying if I posted about it. "That's why you don't do things like this. You just can't trust people."

Feeling warmth on my skin, I got to running. The day was late. These twenty miles weren't going to run themselves.

Highway 40 is a mainline from Vernal, Utah, through Steamboat Springs, Colorado, and over the Rocky Mountains. If you were driving, you'd arrive in Silverthorne at I-70 and take that toward Denver. But also, if you were driving and didn't have business in the quaint mountain village of Steamboat Springs and the ones in between, you wouldn't come this way. The winding highway over the Rocky Mountains added at least an hour between Denver and Salt Lake City when compared to the faster I-80 route through Wyoming. What that meant for me was that the traffic I had experienced coming into Vernal had dissipated. Aside from the occasional semi and Subaru Forester with a "Colorado Native" bumper sticker, it was me, the open road, and a blazing hot sun.

My feet shuffled along the ground, already feeling sore in a worn pair of Asics that needed to go. My shoes were white-and-teal Kayanos, size nine—one of eleven identical pair donated by a running store in Milwaukee.

"Your gait is slightly pronated. That means your ankles collapse in," the store manager had said, showing me with her hands what she meant with her palms flat toward the floor, tilting her thumbs slightly down. She'd watched me run on their in-store treadmill and reported to me her analysis. "This shoe you're in is neutral. I recommend something with more stability."

Until that conversation, I bought whatever pair was on sale. As a young recreational runner who also enjoyed cross-training, it really didn't matter. A three-mile run one day, a four-mile run the next. Push-ups on the ground, balanced sit-ups on a bench. Whether I was in a neutral shoe or a stable one, a flat shoe or a padded one, my body would manage. The distance I ran back then was something it could easily do.

Training to run across the country changed that. Doing it in the wrong shoe could mean not doing it at all after the hours upon hours of the same pressure compounding on my body, multiplied by the year I'd trained and stretched across the 3,288 miles it would take to actually do it. Stress fractures, shin splints, runner's knee, plantar fasciitis, Achilles tendinitis, Iliotibial tendinitis—all the -itises. These are the things people concerned themselves with when they considered what I was doing. Two men attempted a crossing the year before, and one dropped out halfway through. His entire lower leg was bright red—shiny like the color of a cherry, inflamed and unable to heal from the ongoing muscle damage that he inflicted on it by continuing. The cure was rest and ice, ten weeks of it. He hobbled home on a set of crutches.

I stored the eleven pairs of stability shoes fitted for me under the futon couch. Upon unboxing, I'd ink the date across the side of the sole (to tell them apart) and tie my foot into the delightful cradle that was a brand-new running shoe. I thought to do so this morning after I packed the peanut-butter-and-jelly sandwich into the cooler on top of a can of Coca-Cola, but decided instead to squeeze one more run out of this pair. I regretted that decision now.

God, it's hot out here, I breathed heavily, weighed down by the heat, wiping beads of sweat from my brow. The temperature climbed, and I knew that the option to sleep in and run late was gone. Spring was behind me for good. It was early summer, with *real* summer and its triple digits across the Midwest just beyond it. The pavement baked my body from below while the sun bore down overhead, and it was just a taste of what was to come.

It's time to stop messing around, I scolded myself. I had to get myself up earlier, and Nate would have to come with. No excuses. *Now* the event would get real.

I squeezed a warm spray of fruit punch into my mouth and ran on.

The hills rolled in layers, the nearest one being the color of dead grass, the next being a darkish brown, and the last being a hazy blue that melted into a horizon of sky that domed above me. The great blue was unmarked by clouds. The vast plains were unshaded by trees. There was no reprieve until I arrived at the car. Nowhere to be but in the awful, hard here.

I ran past the large highway pullout and the sheds for sale. I ran past the dinky town of Dinosaur and the Welcome Center that Nate and I visited the day before. We had poked around the information boards and dinosaur statues, then gladly took the free "Colorful Colorado" trucker hats the volunteer gave us.

"Are you here to view the canyon area?" the older woman asked. She was a tiny little strong thing with short, curly gray hair underneath a wide-brimmed hat. She wore shorts, tall socks, hiking boots, and a bandanna around her neck. She looked exactly like the kind of person who should welcome people to the state of Colorado.

"We might check it out," I replied. "Right now, we're here because I'm running across America for multiple sclerosis."

"It's just up the road that way," she said, pointing east, grazing over my cross-country comment, excited to talk about the canyon area. "It's very scenic. Which way are you headed?"

"That way," I replied. "East, to New York."

"You'll run right past it then," she said, smiling. "I've been here a bit. I've seen a few of you in my day. You're in much better shape than some of the others."

I smiled in appreciation and also wasn't surprised that she had met others. Unlike her, I hadn't come across transcontinental running until I googled it from the ship in Barcelona. To my amazement, people had been running across America since 1909, with the first woman doing it in 1960. A handful of people were running across the country at any given time, many of them for charity, but none of them raising as much as I said I would. I wasn't deterred.

Well, they're obviously not doing it the right way, I thought of the fundraising, brash and inexperienced. Then I abruptly quit my job and founded a charity.

The woman turned to Nate, "Are you running too?"

"I run sometimes, but not like she's doing," he said. "I manage the logistics and operations."

"Oh?" she said curiously, "What kind of operations?"

"There's a lot that goes into it," I offered quickly. "It's a lot of hours on the road, moving our caravan, setting up. We've got a fundraising event in Denver two weeks from now that he's helping organize."

"Oh." She nodded, thinking about this spattering of information. "Well, stop and see the canyon if you can. It's quite a sight!"

I ran past it now, dragging myself along, not stopping as she suggested. Maybe if I had woken up earlier. Maybe if I had done more than a couple miles by now. Maybe if it wasn't so ungodly hot that I couldn't think about viewing anything except the inside of our cooler for a cold can of Coca-Cola. But I hadn't, I hadn't, and it wasn't.

I hardly noticed the sign that marked the canyon area. A road from its sign went toward a cluster of trees. Beyond that were two plateau shelves, and maybe the canyon was beyond that? Either way, it all seemed very far from where I was. I lumbered past, doing all I could to move forward. I put my head down and pushed on in pursuit of Nate, parked somewhere up ahead.

COLORFUL COLORADO

The road rose up in a slant, tilting toward the mountains. I shuffled up in misery, coaching myself to the next crest.

The car will be just there, I told myself, because the car had always been there. Nate had never gone too far. *Ice-cold Coca-Cola is over that hill.*

Then I'd arrive, and the car wasn't just there. It wasn't just anywhere. It was nowhere. The land was barren, and there was no ice-cold Coca-Cola.

"What the *fuck*?" I said out loud, slowing to a walk. "Where the *fuck* is the car?"

I put my hands on my knees and hung my head. *God, it's hot. Where the fuck is the car?* Looking at my watch, I had been running for over an hour, well past when I'd usually see Nate, which normally would be just fine, except now it wasn't. I had beaten myself up since awaking. It was hotter than I expected, my feet were stuffed into a worn pair of shoes that made it feel like I was barefoot, and now my head felt like it could explode. I felt my heart beat in my face. *Thub. Thub. Thub.*

Standing, I looked behind me at an empty road, squinting again at the omnipresent sun. Ahead, it was the same. I wiped the sweat from my brow. The gritty saltiness of dried sweat felt like sandpaper on my skin.

He has to be up ahead, I told myself. Or had he gone back to the RV and lost track of time? Was he napping? Eating? Sitting in the air conditioning while I melted on the highway? The thought of him doing anything pleasant brought tears to my eyes. Feeling chalky and like the dam might burst, I squeezed the last spray of warm, frothy fruit punch into my mouth. I took a deep breath and let it out slowly.

I would not cry.

Here, at this moment, I hated how much I allowed myself to depend on him. I expected him to be here. He said he would be here. "Just a few miles up the road." He had said, and it had been more than a few miles. So where the fuck was he?

The first two decades of my life, I spent watching my mother need others, like a weak animal burdening the herd, so I clung to everything that neediness wasn't—independence, self-reliance, strength. I would not need my mother because she was sick. I couldn't count on her being there. Her extended hospital stays, her seizures, her MS, they all showed me that. I loved her, but I wouldn't *need* her. And if I couldn't count on her, who could I count on except myself?

Until now, and look.

Considering my options—waiting where I was, walking along, or continuing in a shuffle—I decided to run. I could wait, but why? Without shade, water, or anything to cool myself with, it was just as much agony standing there as it was to move along. He would find me eventually, and until then, I would cover as much ground as I could.

I started again, shuffling along, running toward the mountains when...

She'll be coming 'round the mountain when she comes. (My mind singing in a southern drawl.)
She'll be coming 'round the mountain when she comes.
She'll be coming 'round the mountain
She'll be coming 'round the mountain
She'll be coming 'round the mountain when she comes.
Yeehaw.

The song went around once, then again. It was from my childhood, and I hadn't thought of it in God knows how long, but now here it was, up from the depths. A hundred repetitions later, maybe a thousand? (It was all one too many.) I heard a car behind me. It slowed. Only then, when there was a chance it was him, did I turn to look.

"Babe, where have you been?" he asked, rolling beside me with the window down. I could hear the AC blasting from the front counsel.

"I was going to ask you the same thing," I replied.

"Didn't you see the car? I parked it at the edge of that canyon visitor center."

I looked back in the direction he came. I remembered the sign, but I hardly recalled a building. I never saw the car.

"It was a bit off the road," he said. "But I thought for sure you'd see it."

"Well, I didn't," I said. "Can you pull over and pop the trunk?"

I opened the Coca-Cola from the cooler and took a long pull of the chilled carbonated sugar. It tingled down my throat and into my stomach.

"I thought you would stop," Nate said, coming from the driver's side door. "It was a pretty cool little place. It had dinosaur bones, and I guess the canyon viewing area is just over that range, and–"

"I started too late to stop," I said, cutting him off. "At this rate, I won't be done until dinner."

I sat on the bumper of the trunk, opening my peanut-butter-and-jelly sandwich.

It wasn't necessarily about Nate, but also it wasn't not about him. Wasn't he supposed to be watching out for me? Couldn't he tell how fucking hot it was? How hard was it to follow someone in a car? I was angry for sleeping in, for having to run in the heat, for relying on him—that he veered off the route and enjoyed dinosaur bones while I suffered—at myself for being so stupid, for trusting Spade.

Nate sat down beside me. The car sank lower on the shocks. "You okay?"

"Yeah," I said, not knowing what to say. "It's just really hot, and these shoes are done." The bottoms of my feet ached in a way I hadn't felt since my first marathon. My soles throbbed in pain. Each step I took was a direct impact between the road and my feet carrying the weight of my body. When everything was in sync, the force was absorbed with ease. I'd lean forward into the stride and hit my forefoot. A well-cushioned shoe dispersed the pressure.

Now, wearing these shoes with no miles left on the tread, it felt as if I was beating my feet with a wooden plank. And my form certainly wasn't dialed. I ran fully upright, my shoulders hunching, carrying myself in the only position I could manage to cover the miles, shuffling down the highway, cursing at the world.

"You want to get in the car? We can get new shoes and come back out later?"

"No," I replied. "There's no time. I'll do another six now and eat lunch before the last eight."

"It won't take that long, babe. Just a quick drive up and back," he suggested.

"Nate, there's no time," I snapped. "We can't sleep in *and* view the canyon *and* drive back to the RV whenever I don't feel like being out here *and* get twenty miles done. That's not how this works."

He didn't say anything at first. I didn't look him in the eye.

"Okay," he said, standing from the trunk. "I'll stay on the road."

"Okay," I replied, stuffing the last bit of sandwich into my mouth. I felt like a bitch, but I couldn't help it. Was this a run across America or not?

If I had had any tact or empathy, which I didn't, I could have tried to explain how the miles had come over me. They were there. They always were. And no amount of driving to and from the RV for new shoes would change that.

We could have toured more, I suppose, like we had in Tahoe, had my mind allowed it. There was no one telling me how far I had to run or when I had to be where, except the voice inside my head that reminded me I had said I'd run twenty to thirty miles a day, so that's what I would do. When the running group wanted to meet in Salt Lake City, I did the math according to that average and told them a date. I could have said any date. They didn't care. But I did. Even when a whiteout snowstorm rolled through, making it dangerous to run and nearly impossible to see, I told Nate to drop me on the highway to stay on schedule. When I had to cut that day short, it wasn't a *relief*. I wasn't *relaxed*. All I thought about were the eleven miles that remained and when I'd make them up.

And now I had said I'd be in Denver by June 4 for a fundraising event, so I would. To do that, I'd have to run twenty-one miles a day for the next fourteen days with no room for error, thanks to Spade and the recent vehicle repairs. There was no beautiful balance between running and sightseeing as I dreamed up to him on the cruise ship. This was not that at all. It was only what it was, which was running and fundraising—and a whole hell of a lot of both and nothing else.

And, at the core of me, I *wanted* to run, even when it felt like hell. I wanted to be a person who raised half a million dollars by running across the country. In order to do that, I had to do it. That was it. I never bothered to explain these things. I thought it was obvious.

Running down the highway again, I no longer felt like my head was going to explode. My body had cooled with the water I poured on it, and with it, my temper.

I got this, I thought. *Six now and another eight after lunch.*

In this tempered state, the world, even in its crispiness, offered wonders. Now it was prairie dogs, chirping as they poked up and down from their holes, but there had been other wonders as well—an 80G silver iPod that still worked, a toy light saber, another license plate for the collection.

Each sunrise felt like a real-life watercolor painting, and the land around each bend was new. There were buffalo and llamas. Long-horned cattle and no-horned cattle. Tiny birds and big birds and colorful birds, and every time I saw one, I thought of my mother, who loved birds because, as she said, "They could go wherever they wanted."

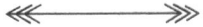

MY FIRST TIME IN Colorado was not during my move to Boulder. It happened in 2006, the summer before my move, when I was a junior in college and I was road-tripping across the country in a powder-blue minivan with my parents and sister, touring graduate schools. We loaded a cooler with ice, canned soda, cold cuts, and cheese into the vehicle before driving as far as we could until someone had to pee.

Because my father couldn't hear well, we didn't listen to the radio. He said that the melody sounded like that character from Charlie Brown named Linus, a string of bumbled *womp-womps* that didn't make sense. Instead, we read books, and we looked out the window. We played "I Spy," and we tried to pet Dad's ear hair while he drove without him noticing that it was us. We laughed until our stomachs hurt. Mom, because of her MS fatigue, mostly slept.

THE LONG RUN HOME

    Our first destination was Flagstaff, Arizona, where I knew quite quickly I didn't want to attend for the silly reason that I didn't like the color of the lab's lime-green tiles. If I were going to spend the next two years of my life in a room, I should enjoy the aesthetics.

    Before heading north to Denver, we stopped to stand on the edge of the Grand Canyon. There, I marveled at the magnitude of the crevasse, though it didn't look real. I stared and stared, knowing that it was before me but feeling also like I was peering at a canvas draped in front of my eyes. To fully understand it, I would need to be in it. I'd have to hike it, feel it beneath my feet, stand at its bottom and look up toward its top, breathe its air, ride its river, camp under its stars. To truly know a thing of its size, both its beauties and miseries, one must be surrounded by it. And no amount of staring at it from the edge can prepare a person for the raw, absolute experience of what it's like to truly be in it.

    From the canyon's edge, we drove to Denver by way of I-70. We toured the campus, then headed to the Rocky Mountain National Park along Highway 34 in Estes Park. Driving the narrow switchbacks, unrestricted by guardrails, my stomach leaped into my throat. The slightest mistake could send our van tumbling top over bottom down a steep, rocky slope. My father steered the vehicle this way, then that, and I gazed out the window in nervous amazement, not knowing that a few years from then, I'd be arriving at its western escarpment on foot, running across the dry, thirsty plains to its west, melting in its unrelenting sun.

    I melted now, running down the highway in the heat until the miles did, melting together one after another until the days did, running until I wasn't to the west of the range, but at it, arriving in Steamboat Springs 129 miles later on my birthday.

    That morning, running miles that matched my age, I began twenty-six miles west of the quaint mountain village. At this distance, though the Rocky Mountains were near, I couldn't see them yet. The land instead came alive with its snowmelt.

    The air felt crisp. A creek at my side gurgled. The atmosphere vibrated. Even if I didn't know what I was to come upon, I could feel it—a monster of a range that extended north to south (from the tip of Canada into New Mexico) as far as I planned to run east to west. I knew the range in some ways when I snowboarded her peaks while living in Colorado, but not like this. Not on the run as I would do now. I told a reporter months ago that I would not run around them, as she suggested, but rather, I would run over them.

She laughed in delight at my response. From afar, I could be a wonder, like watching the power of a freight train from the safe distance of a nearby town. Up close was a different experience. One had to know when to step off the tracks.

Earlier that morning, Nate had given me a gift for my birthday, something that surprised me. I had had no expectations except to be crewed.

"I picked it up in town while you did the interview at the paper." He smiled. "It's not much, but it made me think of you."

The tissue paper inside the gift bag crinkled in my hand. Inside was a book, *Gutsy Girls—Stories of Young Women Who Dare* and a *Runner's World* magazine that featured a shoe-buying guide and nine ways to improve my agility.

"Thank you," I said, feeling grateful. I opened the book and pressed its crease to my nose, inhaling—a habit I had of every book I held. I smelled its bound pages, breathing it in to fully know it.

"Happy birthday!" he said, leaning over the bed for a kiss. His palm pushed down on the mattress, tipping me toward him, and our lips met. Pulling away, he asked, "You want to lounge for a bit? Read?"

I smiled, shaking my head no. "I think I'll run now. We can lounge later."

"Oh, come on. It's your birthday." He pulled at me. "Don't you want to relax?"

My commander pulled too.

"Running can be relaxing," I said, moving from the bed, trying to keep things light. I wanted to run. I always did. I wanted not to have to explain why.

Running along Highway 40, I felt cheerful. Instead of splitting the day's miles, I would run the full distance at once, clearing up the afternoon for Nate and me to stroll around downtown and enjoy the touristy ski town. It was part of my motivation for getting out the door, to complete my miles and enjoy myself, that and the massive burger I'd eat with a cold draft beer to wash it down. The miles rolled on like the lush rolling hills. The fields of brittle, dry grass had transitioned into plains of watered reeds, nourished by the flow of the Yampa River, an unblocked waterway that started in the Rocky Mountains and cascaded through the heart of Steamboat. I danced my feet along the rumble strip, which felt much better now in a new pair of shoes inked with the date I opened them four days prior—May 21.

Before putting them on this morning, I drew smiley faces on the bottom of each of my toes with a black Sharpie to run happy. Nate chuckled at me like one might at a toddler.

For the first time in my life, my birthday wouldn't only be about me. I would do what I wanted to—run—but I'd do it with a purpose. It would be about me *and* my mom, as it had always been—a blend of the day I came into this world mixed with the journey she endured so that I could arrive. She had been tough during my birth, my father told me in my teens, in an effort to show me who she really was.

"The day you were born, when it was time, she just pushed fiercely. I could hear others screaming through the walls. But your mother, she hardly made a noise."

I nodded at him and wondered, because the woman he told me about and the woman I knew were not the same, at least not in the ways that mattered to me at the time. By then, whole days would go by when she could hardly do a thing for herself. Her spirit was strong, but her body had withered. The resentment of what we lost bubbled within me until I screamed at her over something insignificant, like when she offered to help me search for a pen on the cluttered countertop, and instead of taking her offer, I shooed her away and told her she couldn't.

He must have known that it wasn't about her or whatever I screamed about. That it was about what had been taken. That it was about what we'd never get back. Unjust festering within until I erupted.

I thought of that version of myself often while I ran, as I did now. I was so mad then.

Out here doing this, I already knew. What I had felt had already changed.

When I stepped off the cruise ship and into this role, part of me cooled with the solution I had been given. Running across the country felt as big to me as the disease itself. Flying home from Miami, sitting on an aircraft in seat 12A, and arriving in Milwaukee, I peered out the egg-shaped window down at the cold earth blanketed in dingy, blanched snow. I traded sunny palm trees for bare maple limbs reaching toward an overcast sky like nerve endings and felt relieved. I stared at the neat plots of city land framed by charcoal roads painted with yellow lines. The roads were an endless tic-tac-toe grid spread out for miles. Miles and miles. All of the miles. I would run them here in any direction I chose, and that was powerful. I would do it for her. I would do it for myself. I would do it because I could.

In between training runs and building the charity, I'd take my mom out to Starbucks, for a pedicure, or for a drive underneath a canopy of trees. I'd come home from teaching my 9:00 a.m. fitness class, and there she'd be, sitting on the couch.

"You want to get cleaned up?" I asked, sitting down next to her on a cream-colored couch covered in washed-out stains that came from eating lunch on it with her adult hands that don't quite cooperate.

"Sure." She smiled.

I stood and took her under the arm, as my father had done for years, and helped her up. Once upright, we made our way through the kitchen, over the exposed subfloor—a renovation project my father never finished—and around a five-gallon bucket filled with wrappers. Upstairs in the full bath, I closed the toilet lid and sat her down.

I pushed up my sleeves.

In the shower, I placed her seat—a metal-and-canvas foldable camp chair and then turned on the water to warm it. Kneeling at her feet, I removed her slip-on Dr. Scholl's shoes that supported her balance and didn't require her to tie laces. I pulled off her socks, her elastic waistband pants, her Praise Jesus top, and her elastic bra and panties. Fully naked, I supported her weight as she stood and held the wall to enter the soaking tub. Her leg lifted over the heightened edge with the fluidity of an unoiled Tin Man. I held her and helped her sit under the water.

Squeezing shampoo into my open palm, I lathered her hair, not holding my breath as my younger self had once done. I breathed in fully. I was here. I was happy to help. I cleaned her while I cleansed myself.

Once dressed, I dried her chin-length hair with a towel, then a hair dryer. I curled the ends, and then I rubbed foundation on her face. I brushed blush across her cheeks. Then I swept mascara upon her lashes. My father was a saint for the way he fed and washed her daily, but these touches of femininity were abandoned when she could no longer do them herself. Her legs were pale and hairy, her hair was a short bob she never preferred, and her clothes were pull-on. Everything was practical.

Here, though, in this moment, I didn't want her to feel practical. I wanted her to feel special.

"There," I said, looking at her face. "How does that feel?"

"That feels nice," she said. Her eyes twinkled. "I'm glad you're home."

I looked at her and smiled. "Me too," I replied. It felt profound that I meant it.

Running toward Steamboat, I was no longer home with her, but I still was. I ran toward the rocky peaks, thinking of these moments, thinking of us, thinking of what it meant to be twenty-six years old and to have wasted so much time not doing this work. There was much to do. It was a relief that I started.

Four miles outside of the mountain village, my hips felt sore. Recent weeks had been packed with twenty milers, twenty-two milers, and twenty-five milers back-to-back-to-back. It wasn't the distance that wore at my muscles on this day. It was doing them all at once. I ran with a stiff gait toward the car. It was my last crew stop before finishing a marathon distance on the west edge of town.

"How you doing?" Nate asked. He stood next to an open trunk.

"Sore," I replied. "I'm ready to be done."

"Want to stop? We can come back here tomorrow."

"Nah," I said. "I can do it. It's just uncomfortable. Best to get it done."

"I figured." He smiled. "We got a message just a bit ago from Bert. He can meet us over his lunch to help us park at the condo."

"Oh, cool!" I said. Bert was the friend of a friend from Denver, and our free stay in Steamboat. We hadn't met yet, but we'd be staying at his place for two nights. I sat on the bumper with a bag of salt-and-vinegar chips in my hand. "We'll need to dump first, right?"

"Yeah, I think the tanks need it." He agreed. "I checked the map. There's an RV park on this side of town. We can dump the tanks and fill with fresh water, then call Bert at his work number." To us, it was another day. To the world, it was Tuesday.

"Sounds like a plan." I grabbed another chip.

Though my hips were sore and I was ready to be done for the day, I was content. It was beautiful—a sunny day in the high sixties. The air felt cool, as air at elevation does, but it was pleasant with a touch of warmth. The vegetation was lively, the birds danced among the trees, and the breeze came across my salty skin. With Nate at my side and moments like these, what more could I ask for?

"Okay," I said, standing from the frame. "I'll get moving so we can be done for today. Four more miles."

"Four more miles," Nate echoed. "You got this!"

"Thanks!" I shouted back, already on the move. I ran awkwardly, waiting for my hips to loosen. Even sitting for just a few minutes caused my muscles to stiffen. My entire backside, from my hamstrings to my midback, ached. My joints throbbed. My hip flexors pounded.

One mile later, I was more fluid. Pained but fluid. I endured it in an upbeat state, knowing better than to wish it away.

An hour later, we drove the RV into the Steamboat Springs KOA, a picturesque campground sandwiched between the highway and river. The sites were shaded by lush oaks and backed up against a flowing Yampa River. There was a pool, a mini golf course, and a wooden planked bridge that crossed the water to a recreation path on the other side. Standing there, one could see an unobstructed view of Mt. Werner to the east. I was excited to meet Bert, but looking around, I wanted to stay here. I'd park the vehicles and never leave.

The motorhome sat next to the KOA dumping station—a cement pad with a hole in the ground to place the sewer hose. The storage compartment where we stored our sewer hose was directly below a sponsor's tagline on the vinyl wrapping: "Live The Dream" was written directly above our shit-hose compartment. I looked at it on days that I dumped the tanks and chuckled. Some days, living your dream meant dealing with some shit.

While Nate filled the freshwater tank, I walked around the campground, stopping to stand on the planked wooden bridge that crossed the waterway. A pair of kayakers bobbed down the rushing rapids in their bright little boats, and I felt an unexpected pang of jealousy. I waved at them as they passed underneath me, and they waved back. I wondered where they lived. I wondered if it was in a house. I wondered if they loved it as much as I imagined I would, living in this blissful little town nestled in the mountains.

Maybe we'll live here, I thought of Nate and me.

Where we would settle after the run, when we would get married, and where and how we would pay for it were all topics of conversation recently. We daydreamed about our future in the cracks of the running regime, imagining the best place for both of us as we built a life together.

"You're going to love Denver," I sold him. "It's the perfect place, just on the edge of the mountains and close to the airport for travel. It's sunny all the time, it's hot in the summer, and the winters are very manageable. It's nothing like what you experienced in Wisconsin."

As a southern Australian who loved the beach, his arrival in my home state in November didn't exactly fulfill his dreams. It took him an hour and a half to shovel the driveway when it snowed (often), and the one time I let him drive, he hit a patch of ice on a downhill and put my car in the ditch.

COLORFUL COLORADO

The best of what Wisconsin had to offer emerged precisely when we left for San Francisco. It started with the Brewers' spring training and extended all the way to Thanksgiving. It was tailgating and brats. Clear, bright skies. Fresh air, singing birds, and melting snow. It was bubbling summer days at the lake and cooling off in the fresh water. It was cabins up north, a summer evening concert, beer. Spring in Wisconsin, and everything that comes after, is a rebirth each year—for the animals, for the land, for us.

There were things I loved about it, especially my family, but still, I wasn't planning to settle there. It wasn't just a dream for me to move back to Colorado. I made plans for it. When the IRS 501(c)3 application asked for the location of the charity, I penned "Colorado" on the line without hesitation. I would build the charity here near the mountains. It was a fitness-crazed community with intoxicating views and outdoorsy athletes—the kind of people who liked to go kayaking down a river on a Tuesday afternoon. I was this kind of people. Now that Nate and I had a future together, I willed him to be the same.

"There are a bunch of Aussies in Denver. I looked it up." He had let me know. "There's a group on Facebook that gets together to play Aussie rules. They have a practice match while we're in town. I thought I'd swing by."

"Fun," I said.

I watched the backside of the kayakers float down the river now, thinking about it, how perfect it was—that we would do this together and live in Denver afterward. His voice broke me from my daze.

"Ashley! Babe," he called for me, "we're all set. Let's go."

CHAPTER THIRTEEN
Tough Act to Follow

WE MET BERT AT his condo, where he handed us a key. "This is my spare that you can use while you're in town," he said, handing over the notched piece of metal. "I'm not here much, so I won't be around to let you in."

"Thanks," I said, taking it from his hand. "If you're not here," I wondered, looking at his picturesque mountain condo cut into a mound of rising earth, "where are you?"

"Into the mountains, biking mostly," he replied. "And work, of course. But everyone there is an athlete as well, so we get our work done and take off. The office is dead at lunch. Everyone's outside."

I shook my head knowingly. Jealous. It was my ideal life—working to live in the mountains, a granola bar and an apple as my lunch, nimbly carried up the tallest ridge in my trail running pack.

"So, how are you celebrating your birthday?" Bert asked. He held his dirty bike upright at his side in a way that made me know that he was rarely without it. It fit him like my shoes fit me.

"You're looking at it." I smiled, gesturing with my hands. "Twenty-six miles done, and now I'm looking for an excellent burger. Any recommendations?"

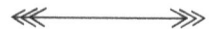

TOUGH ACT TO FOLLOW

NATE AND I SAT bellied up to the bar at an old western eatery downtown across from the Yampa River. The interior was rustic wood and dark metals, with moose heads and bicycles fastened to its walls. This place, like Bert, was all about biking and mountain living. We looked over the menu and placed an order, then drank our draft amber ales while the food cooked.

"Twenty-six, huh?" Nate said. "You're still just a baby."

"Ha!" I blurted, "Hardly. I'm behind." My fingers turned the beer glass around. I watched tiny bubbles rise. "I feel like I should have done this sooner."

"Sooner?" He looked at me, wrinkling his brow. "Like when?"

"I dunno." I shrugged. "It just feels like I should have been doing this all along. That's all."

"Well, you're doing it now, babe. That's more than most people can say."

It was a weekday afternoon in Steamboat Springs, and the restaurant was alive with chatter. Voices hummed through the air. Forks clanged on ceramic plates. Beer gurgled from the tap into chilled pints.

"You know," I said, "I bet we can find a runner to do this every year for the charity."

"Do what?" Nate asked.

"Run across America," I replied. "People do it all the time. We could set it up as a fundraising event to help people with MS. I mean, can you imagine if I had been able to leave the cruise ship and just step into this already set up?"

"Babe, you're not even halfway across. Can we just focus on that? How would we even find someone else to do it? How much money would they have to raise to make it worth it?"

Just then, the barkeep approached us with our burgers. "The American with cheddar, cooked medium," he said, setting the plate down in front of Nate. "And black and blue for the runner, medium rare."

The smell of the cooked beef and fried potatoes wafted to my face. My mouth watered.

"So, she's running across America," the barkeep said to Nate. "But how 'bout you? You're just driving?"

While placing our order, we had talked about why we were in town—that it was my birthday, that I was running across America for my mom.

I reached for the glass ketchup bottle, twisted the cap, and tipped it upside down next to my fries while Nate explained that he helped with logistics and operations.

The barkeep, middle-aged and overweight, let out a low whistle. "That's a tough act to follow, son."

I furrowed my brow. "How so?" I asked. "If it were the other way around, him running and me helping, would he be a tough act for me to follow?"

The man cleared his throat and looked at me, then picked up his bar rag. "Order up," he said and walked away toward the kitchen without replying.

Later, after we had eaten, Nate grabbed my hand on the way out. "Hey. How about I run tomorrow's miles? Let's make this a relay. A real team event! We can cover the distance faster and make more time for fundraising."

"Nate," I replied.

"Ashley, it doesn't matter if you do all the running. We're out here for the cause. We'll bring more awareness if we do it together!"

"I'm not relaying," I said, stopping on the sidewalk to look him in the face. First, he asked in Nevada, then again in Utah. Now, in Colorado. I was tired of him even mentioning it.

What didn't he get? Who cared about someone who started a solo crossing and then decided to relay instead? And really, was it about the fundraising? No explaining about logistics and operations by either of us would change what was—that he was a guy following along in the shadow of a girl's run. It was a dynamic we hadn't considered needed discussion.

"Don't ask again," I told him with conviction.

Arriving at the car, Nate got in and pulled the driver's door shut hard. Was that intentional? Was there tension? And why? I'm only doing what I said I would.

It was so subtle that it was hard to tell. Maybe even, I just imagined it.

TOUGH ACT TO FOLLOW

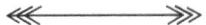

TWO DAYS LATER, I ran up Rabbit Ears Pass, a steep mountain pitch that went toward the sky for seven miles. After the Sierra and Wasatch mountain ranges, the relentless peaks across Nevada, and the 1,203 miles behind me, my body was ready.

I took the incline and felt nimble, like the mountain lions that roamed the dense forest beyond the highway. For ninety minutes, I pumped and exhaled my way to the top, past views of the wet valley below and mounds of dirty, crusted snow clinging to the road's edge, and kept running.

On I ran, crossing the Continental Divide, then past grassy meadows of big-horned sheep and ranches of grazing cows. Past chimney rock and a tiny pond where two boys played with their dog. Past clusters of metal yard art and snowcapped peaks and an orange construction cone that Nate called a "witch's hat." I went until the Rocky Mountains were no longer a place I was running to; I was in them, I was on them, I was running over them.

I ran and ran. When I felt lonely—though I was not alone—I walked. I reached for my phone and called home.

"Hey, how are you?" my sister April said, picking up her phone.

"Good," I replied, not mentioning that I felt lonely. "How are you?"

"Good! *Where* are you?"

"Running through the Rocky Mountains, almost to Silverthorne," I said. I was moving along Highway 9 past Green Mountain Reservoir, twenty-three miles west of I-70. "There's a huge reservoir, people boating. It's pretty amazing."

Overhead, a giant bird glided through the air, circling above the water where the boaters buzzed around. I heard the people's laughter, their faint, happy music floating to me on a gentle breeze. Others gathered at the water's edge. I saw them grilling, drinking. It wasn't until then that I realized it was Memorial Day weekend. People were with their families. Alone on a highway, running another marathon through the mountains, I had nearly forgotten.

"You always did love Colorado," she said. "Are you so excited to be there?"

"Yeah, it's great. It's hard to believe I've run here," I replied. Gravel crunched beneath my shoes. "It'll be better once I get to Denver and see some familiar faces. I really miss you guys. I miss home."

"Aw. We miss you too," she replied, keeping her tone light. "Dad's mowing the lawn, per usual. And I'm sitting with Mom out front. She's watching the birds."

"Lame," I said, picturing it all so perfectly that it made my chest hurt.

"Right? We'll just have some beers and grill out. You know, the same. How about you? What are you two up to?"

Nate was parked somewhere up ahead. For lunch, we'd stop at the campground just north of the reservoir, probably nap, then come back out for nine more miles before dinner. It was "the same" here too, I supposed.

"Running," I replied, "Five more days of it, and then I get a few days off in Denver. Our fundraising event there is on the Fourth."

"Lame," she replied.

I smiled.

"You want to say hi to Mom?" she asked.

"Sure. How's she doing today?"

"Not bad. Not sure what you'll get out of her, but you know how it is. She'll just be happy someone called."

Brain fog and cognitive dysfunction were two of my mother's prominent MS symptoms. She was clever and smart–something I knew more than I witnessed. Oftentimes, what she wanted to say disappeared, like a plume of smoke into the great open air. You could see in her eyes when it happened. Whatever it was was lost somewhere along the highway of her mind. It made having a conversation with her a challenge.

"Hello," I heard her shaky and feeble voice say.

"Hi, Mom. It's Ashley. How are you?" I asked.

"Good. Just, uh, you know... watching... um, uh... the birds."

She sounded tiny. *She*, though, was anything but. To understand the truth of that, you'd have to be with her.

"Me too," I said. "There's a bird flying overhead. It's huge. I'm in Colorado."

"Neat!"

"Yeah, it's really nice. I can see the mountains ahead. They still have snow on them. And I'm almost to Denver. Our fundraising event there is next Wednesday."

Just then, I heard some rustling and an "oop."

Click.

The line was dead.

I sighed and took a drink from my water bottle. My phone rang.

"Hey," I said, picking up.

"Hey, sorry, she dropped the phone," April said.

"Yeah, I know." Sporadic muscle tremors in her hands from MS made holding objects difficult. "I'll say goodbye. I've gotta get moving."

"Okay, I'll hold the phone."

In the muffled background, I could hear April say, "No, I'll hold it." Like one would to a toddler, simple and direct, the way that we were sometimes forced to be with her.

"Ashbee?" Mom said.

"Hey, Mom, I gotta get running, but I just wanted to say I love you, and I miss you."

"Me too, honey. I love you. God bless."

I tucked my phone into its holder.

So what if I was out here on a holiday? So what if I was lonely? *You get to do this*, I reminded myself.

Too easily, I had let my discomfort take my attention. I was reminded of a moment one year prior when I worked as a fitness instructor while building the charity and training for the event. That morning, in particular, I instructed the group of women to meet me at the beach so we could take our workout to the sand to surprise their muscles into pain and growth.

It was humid, it was July, and the sun was relentless. Skin shimmered in a thick layer of sweat under drenched workout tops. I coached my clients the same way I coached myself, with little mercy.

"Three... two... one," I counted down. They dropped to their mats, done with the last set of push-ups at the end of an hour-long class.

Nearby, my mother sat by the group of sweaty women in a red foldable camp chair and smiled, as she often did for no reason at all, watching the low waves lap at the shoreline. I had brought her along—to get her out of the house, to give my dad a few hours alone.

A cluster of seagulls along the beach fought over loose food remains from the day before. The air, though humid, smelled of fresh lake water.

"Jill," a client said, out of breath and resting on her mat. "I'll tell ya, that chair looks nice."

My mother looked at her kindly. "I'll trade places with you."

Like my client, momentary suffering got the best of me. And just as she had done then, my mother helped me refocus.

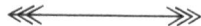

RUNNING AGAIN ON HIGHWAY 9 past the reservoir. I accomplished the remaining miles at a quick pace after the enlightening phone call with my mother, and Nate set up the motorhome at our campsite. He attached the water hose to the spigot, plugged in the electrical and tested the outlets, checked the holding tanks, bled the air from the faucet lines, and set up everything we tucked away while the vehicle was in motion—the blender, the plants, the soaps, and a conglomerate of jars, bottles and food that jostled around in the refrigerator as we drove along, that then tumbled out like a mass of clothes from a dryer when we opened the refrigerator door. I walked up to the site, not far from the highway where I ran, just as he completed this tedious process.

"Stupid fucking antenna," he said under his breath. Inside the RV, he stood near the driving quarters, working an antenna crank that was fixed to the roof.

"That thing's worthless," I said, coming into the main cabin and going toward the fridge. "We should have pulled that TV when we had the chance."

The 1994 box screen I spoke of was fixed into the dash. It was fifteen inches across and three feet deep of usable storage space, had the pointless contraption been pulled from the dash like I had wanted to do before we left. Nate petitioned to keep it, just in case.

At the fridge, I pulled out the sliced turkey, cheddar cheese, lettuce, mayonnaise, and a cold Coca-Cola. From the cupboard above the sink, I grabbed the bread and an unopened bag of salt-and-vinegar chips. The plates were found above the stove, and the cutting board was set across the sink for extra counter space. I placed all these things out and started to assemble my lunch. I looked out the window at a bluebird sky above the mountains.

Nate huffed and cranked. Fiddled and then cranked again.

"Nate, it's just TV."

"I just want *one* thing to be easy," he yelled. Then he slammed his fist against the plush captain's chair across from the couch and stormed out. The door banged closed with a *whack*.

I stared at the static door, then took a bite of my turkey sandwich, and sat down at the dinette to eat.

He wasn't entirely off—not much we had done since leaving Wisconsin would be considered easy. We moved every few days and were limited to showers in tight plastic stalls, confined by both hot water and space. We'd arrive at camp and set up, only to realize we forgot to get propane, something we needed for cooking, warm water, and heat. The propane tank was in-house, meaning we needed the motorhome next to a fill station to get it, meaning we'd have to tear down camp and drive somewhere to do it. But first, we'd need to call to make sure the propane fill station was open. It wasn't like getting gas for the car—we needed the assistance of a certified propane gas operator.

To do anything took nearly eleven steps. As we went along, things broke down—little things like the electrical hot water heater, which we'd been meaning to get fixed, but that was tough to coordinate—it being summer and service centers being booked full and us always moving ninety miles up the road every three days.

At night, washing my face, I'd hunch over a sink no larger than a salad bowl before reaching overhead to turn off the plastic light just feet from my head. Its switch was plastic. The salad bowl sink was plastic. The countertop was not plastic but something just as airy—composite wood that bubbled at the edges from years of water absorption. Even the walls were oddly nomadic.

"Nate," I said one night from the bed, "I can hear the game." He sat on the futon couch, watching a match of Aussie rules football online.

"Babe, it's down as far as it'll go. My earbuds are in the car. It's almost done."

Right, I thought. When is football ever "almost done"?

I huffed and pulled a pillow over my ears, needing to sleep for the next day's marathon.

The outlets worked only when we were plugged into a shoreline or we started the generator, an engine below the couch that sounded like a tractor. The faucets flowed only when we were hooked up to a spigot or when it was pumped from the water tank—a system, too, that had a noise. The furnace warmed only when we had enough propane. The AC cooled only when it had enough wattage.

To do anything was a process. A tedious, noisy process. The road like this—with its sunrise mornings, always moving, tiny spaces, and zero autonomy—was impossible to predict, except if I had asked someone, which I didn't. Half of our team's stamina to endure it was waning, and 128 days of it remained.

Yet, despite it all, I was home.

We were compact and nimble. Mobile and free. Less was more, and I loved it.

On the road running before dawn, I witnessed magnificent rays break the line of a new day, day after day. The sky lit up in a cascade of colors, and I, tiny beneath it, moved along in a sweaty glow. At times, my body hurt, but that's because I used it. We were fed, we were cared for, and in quiet moments among nature, I knew we were watched over as well. This stillness was a birthright—one that I only forgot about when I thought too far ahead. And how fruitless that would be, after all I had learned from my parents.

And so I breathed in the moments, even lonely ones, on the side of the highway. Because this, I knew—it would all pass.

Nate lived this as well, I learned during our months of dating and year-long distance phone calls. He was the one who handed me *The Secret,* a book that shifted everything into motion.

Its pages contextualized things my parents and their faith had been teaching me all along, that my thoughts held power. "If you have faith as tiny as a mustard seed," my father would say, holding his fingers together very closely, quoting the Bible, "you can move mountains. That's how important faith is. If you can think it and believe it, consider it done."

And so I imagined this run into fruition. I believed it to be there, and it came to life.

Nate was the type of person who would give me a book about positive mindset *and* believe in its power, so I had a hard time seeing why he was so wound up over the TV antenna, or me not changing this into a relay run, or him being the driver?

I stared blankly out the window, thinking these thoughts while eating through the entire bag of salt-and-vinegar chips. When it was empty, I licked the seasoning from my fingers and opened my laptop. My fingers typed "RV tow dolly Denver, CO," and hit Search. As I scrolled through hundreds of dollars' worth of products I didn't think we needed, I reminded myself that everything didn't have to be my way.

Relationships are about compromise, I told myself. *This will help bring him ease.*

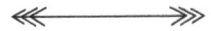

EASE, THOUGH, WAS NOT my focus, so two days later, when I hit the sharp, nine-mile incline of Loveland Pass and my muscles burned in a way I hadn't felt yet, a smirk came across my face, and I leaned in.

Finally.

Green Mountain Reservoir had come and gone. I ran through Dillon and underneath I-70 to the ascent I was on now, toward the tallest point of the whole run. A monster of a summit lay between Denver and me. It was 11,990 feet of mountain called Sinktau, and I wasn't far from where I left its base. To get there, I'd climb 2,650 feet.

Less than an hour prior, Nate had pulled into a closed Keystone ski parking area and dropped me off.

"Here we go, babe. You ready for this?" he said, looking toward the top beyond a gigantic wall of pines. We couldn't see its peak, but the challenge of running there pulled at me. The air felt crisp and different, void of oxygen. My path was sharp and rising.

"You bet," I replied. I was ready.

Running it now, I realized I wasn't ready, at least not in the way I had imagined—light and nimble like the mountain lion I had been on Rabbit Ears. The ache of a hollowing atmosphere and the effort to move in spite of it crushed my pretense of lightness. The chilled air nipping at my lungs. Desperate for oxygen, my muscles pulsed in misery. Driving my limbs and forcing my breath, I moved at a labored pace.

Yes, I pressed. *Bring it.*

Ahead and above me, an eighteen-wheeler hammered an engine brake. I couldn't see it, but I could hear it around the switchback where the pavement cut up to the left, so I checked behind me and crossed the road for safety. Thirty seconds later, it glided down west on Highway 6 in a *whoosh,* and with it, the branches of evergreens tousled in its stream. They lined the road, a dense gathering of pines, towering like frosted gods with mounds of snow at their feet. A critter scurried up a trunk to my left. A trickle of snow melt babbled down on my right. I pushed on and suffered in between— drawing for breath, forcing it out, driving my thundering heart.

Up I went, passed occasionally by a hazardous rig routed from the Eisenhower Tunnel and cyclists who sought this same twisted pleasure.

"You got it," a biker would say, heading up, winded as they pumped back and forth on their geared machine.

"You too," I'd breathe out, watching them go. We were kin; they were here for it too—to mute the world for just a moment in the consumption of harmless suffering.

Eyes down, my mind said. *Focus on the road.*

And so I did, locking my gaze on the line. My peripheral morphed into a blur of color blocks in motion.

If you don't look up, there is no up. The ground is flat. And I believed myself. *The ground is flat*, I repeated to myself. *The ground is flat.*

Minutes later, my breathing calmed.

Up I went, fabricating my way past Arapahoe Basin and its side-country skiers. Trickles of melt turned into modest mountain waterfalls, and mounds of snow became full banks of it taller than me. The pines dwindled, refusing to grow where living things could not, and I pressed on, running, then hiking, then running, then hiking, then running—as if underwater and breathing through a straw.

My lungs ached. My muscles throbbed. My whole body pleaded with me to stop.

I refused.

Running a switchback, I looked out at a stretch of stunning mountain peaks that went on for miles, far beyond what I could see. The raw beauty of the range at this height was powerful; it stilled me in my place.

What a dazzling place, this earth. I heard from within.

I marveled at the truth. I could not disagree.

Peaks jutted to my left, and my sight followed them, snow-covered and gleaming in the sunlight. Below me, another biker ascended on the road past the ski basin. Looking up, beyond where I stood, the highway snaked this way, then that, and finally to the summit.

Get there first came the next instructions.

And taking off in a run, I listened.

My heart open, my body working, my mind bending the world of its inclines—that's how I overcame Loveland Pass. That's how I arrived at its base in the first place.

CHAPTER FOURTEEN
Just Visiting

"**SO, HOW MANY MARATHONS** have you done?" Steve asked, running by my side.

He worked the accounting for a Denver marathon training group who was following my run online—except now I was close enough to Denver, and they could join in person. Steve was the first of a number of runners lined up to meet me throughout the next several days. The training group owner, David, had emailed me months ago.

"When are you coming through?" he wrote. "We paced Blue Planet when they ran through Denver a few years ago, and we'd love to do the same for you!"

I didn't know what Blue Planet was or how David found my run, but he did more than line up pacers. The moment I crossed the state line, he connected me with hosts and businesses all across Colorado. My new hydration pack, Climacool sweat-wicking tops for summer, and Merrell wool running socks were all gifted to me thanks to David's support.

"Official marathon races?" I responded to Steve's question, striding downhill with ease.

"Yeah."

"Just one," I answered.

He let out a burst of laughter. "This is crazy."

Running at his side, I throttled my pace, not because he was slow, but because I was coasting down from a mountaintop and giddy with the company. He and I were covering nineteen miles together—the most I had run with a person since I'd left San Francisco. Steve was a marathoner, logging his long training run with me to keep me company. It was a Wednesday morning, and he adjusted his work schedule to cover the miles with me. The fact that he wanted to run this much and intentionally rearranged his day to accommodate it gave me a sense of kinship. We were both out here because we wanted to be, propelled by a motive we didn't have to explain to each other.

"I've done a handful of marathons and still can't fathom the kind of miles you're doing every day," he said. "And you look perfectly healthy. How is that possible?"

We talked and ran—glided, really—along a frontage road in the valley of two mountain peaks that were covered with giant pines and exposed rock faces. The path paralleled and occasionally crossed the interstate, under or atop, where cars, SUVs, and semis buzzed back and forth in fast, neat lines.

In spots along the frontage road, a recreation path would appear, and when it did, we'd run along that until it ended or turned into a tiny sidewalk, as it did in the small town of Silver Plume. That's when Steve told me there was a big push by local residents to have the recreation path extend all the way from the Loveland Ski area to Golden, a city at the foothills of the mountains where I'd be in a few days' time.

"It's been constructed in sections, but residents want pedestrian access the whole way. That area just north of where we met is new." It sounded exactly like the kind of thing Colorado residents would push for.

The miles passed quickly, and along the way, I learned that the DOT shut down a whole lane of I-70 for the record-breaking cross-country attempt by Marshall Ulrich two years prior. Marshall was an ultrarunner and mountaineer from Idaho Springs, a town up ahead that was our finishing point for the day. "The King of Ultra," *Outside Magazine* called him. His name came up to me a handful of times while I prepared for my crossing, mostly while running fifty-mile trail races.

"You should watch his documentary," a middle-aged, burly man said at one race.

I'd responded that I would, letting the man talk about Marshall in a grandiose, godlike way while having no intention of watching a documentary of someone else's run across America until I had completed my own. Witnessing his obstacles, even if he overcame them, while I attempted to navigate my own, could have consequences I wasn't interested in entertaining.

Later, I'd read that running along the interstate saved Marshall nine miles in distance versus my route up Highway 6 over Loveland Pass. Running through the rustic downtown streets of Georgetown with Steve at my side, talking about all things running—gear and races and the like, I decided I was happy to do it my way.

The nine-mile difference came from two massive holes a team of men bored through the heart of the mountain in 1973 and 1979 to finish the interstate highway system. The Eisenhower Tunnel was 1.6 miles through, rather than switchbacked up and over, and exited toward the town of Dillon on the west side.

That's where I was three days ago, running along Highway 9 past the Green Mountain Reservoir, when the sight of I-70 brought tears suddenly to my eyes. I had taken its path many times before, up it and back, on the days I broke away from work to escape into the mountains with my snowboard. Its familiarity—the gas station I'd fill up at, the sports shop where I bought goggles, the brewery where I ate fries—swelled emotion in my throat.

That I would experience this and yet have little empathy for Nate's emerging discontent was a product of our conversations. I wondered if he missed home—what it must be like to do this while his family and friends were on a different day of the week altogether. And then I reminded myself that we had already talked about it, that he said it'd be okay, that these few months were only the beginning of a lifetime away from his family. I chose to believe the version of what we thought would happen rather than the one that was actually happening.

"If we're going to be together, you'll need to move to America," I whispered to him over the phone one summer evening while we daydreamed about the run and what our life together could be like. "I can't live that far from my family." When discussing things like leaving a continent to be with someone, it's best to be honest, forward. It came naturally to me anyway, as these were ways I had always been.

"I love America," he whispered in return. "And, more importantly, babe, I love you."

I cooed back into the phone, smiling, floating. He'd move to America to be with me. How perfectly romantic. It seemed clear, settled. Like a pair of young teenagers passing notes in class, love, we thought, was all we'd need.

Approaching Nate at the car parked in a gravel pullout along the frontage road, love wasn't all I needed anymore. I needed that and also a bag of salt-and-vinegar chips, a refill of my water bottle, a banana, and a swig of Coca-Cola, preferably chilled, still in the can. He knew these things already and got to it, taking my water bottle from me and filling it with ice and water before scooping my fruit-punch-flavored hydration mix into the open top. I took a bite of a banana. Steve stood with us, chatting away.

"You know, this is pretty cool," he commented, unscrewing the top of his own handheld water bottle. "Maybe I would run a couple marathons in a row if I had someone filling up my drink and bringing me food."

I smiled at Nate. "Yeah, he does a great job. This would be a lot of work without him."

"Ah, don't give her any ideas, Steve," Nate joked. "She's already fantasizing about helping someone else do it."

"Really?" Steve looked at me. "You'd want to do this again?"

"Well, not *me*," I said, digging my hand into the chip bag. "But people run across America all the time. I'm just thinking it'd be cool if I could help someone do it with the resources I've built in exchange for fundraising."

"Huh," Steve said, thinking. "Well, I'd never do the whole thing, but maybe a week. You know, like a vacation from work or something."

I crunched the chips in my mouth and considered his comment. "How much would you fundraise?" I asked.

"Nothing." Steve laughed. "I'm more of a giver. Asking people for money isn't my thing."

"Weak," I joked back. "You can't get something for nothing."

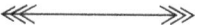

A FEW DAYS LATER, the state's capital emerged like Oz's Emerald City through the motorhome's windshield, soaring and majestic like I hadn't remembered it. It felt big, though it really wasn't, at least not in the same way that New York was, or Chicago, or the Emerald City in *The Wizard of Oz* when the twinkling green towers emerged to Dorothy over the horizon like a city of magic she had only dreamed of.

It was big in ways that mattered only to me—big because of how I had become more of myself in the nine months that I had lived here. I was who I was today, someone who felt sure enough to leave a dream job to pursue a charity run across America and was now actually doing it, in part because of the risks I took to live here, in part because of the ones I took while living here.

Denver was "mile high" at 5,280 feet above sea level, but that hardly felt possible after all the driving down we had done to get there. I led our caravan of two, me in the camper with Nate following behind in the car, as we did when we moved camp. I hardly asked which one he cared to drive. I just took the keys to the big one and went.

Down we drove—down from where I ran above the tree line and could hardly breathe, down from where we slept the night before along a frontage road pullout after my run with Steve (where I closed my eyes and drifted to sleep to the sound of a rushing river), down from the quaint mountain towns littered with both grand homes and modest ones, down past Red Rocks at Morrison where I popped my ears for the last time on the descent.

"You're not supposed to do that," I imagined Nate telling me. "Move your jaw instead."

I put my hand to my nose and blew the pressure out anyway, feeling relief before placing my hand back upon the steering wheel, safely at ten and two.

Passenger cars whipped past me on the left, and I held the

motorhome at a fluctuating sixty miles per hour to the right. I pulsed my foot up and down on the brake, as my father had told me to, so the brakes wouldn't fail.

"You'll see sand and gravel runaway ramps throughout the mountains," he said. "You won't need those if you pulse the brakes."

I did as he said while at the same time imagining what it would be like if I did it wrong—picturing the breaks giving way and the vehicle gaining speed, me having to maintain control while whipping around vehicles between the cement barrier and rocky mountain face, the runaway ramp appearing, steering into it, knowing that stopping would come only after I slammed the motorhome into a mound earth at who knows what speed.

In the driver's seat now, I drove on, imagining the worst that could happen while also hoping it wouldn't, trusting myself if it did. It was a lot like running along busy highways, a lot like starting a nonprofit business. Much out of my control could go wrong, and I just carried on as if it would go right.

Denver, a familiar sight, up ahead.

I looked at its cluster of Tetris block buildings erupting from an otherwise flat ground that spread out in every direction except to the west. There, at my back, were the big peaks, and those were behind me now, so I thought. Seeing flatness for the first time in weeks rather than a canvas of snow-covered ridges, I imagined the Midwest plains ahead and open stretches of level highway—a happy flat glide into Wisconsin. From here, I'd run home. It felt poetic.

At a third of the way across the country, Denver was my first personal milestone. To make it this far was an obvious indicator of both my abilities as a runner and also a tangible marker of my progress. A mile could drag on forever while actually running it, but arriving here made it clear to me that a thousand of them were behind me, and the two thousand that were ahead would come and go too. Before long, I'd be in New York.

Driving through the playground city that I loved—a place where the person that I was more closely resembled the one Nate fell in love with—I was reminded of who I had been here, testing the boundaries of identities without any mind of consequence: the chill snowboarder, the polished waitress, the fitness junkie, the drug and booze-fueled bargoer. Now that I had run here for a charity I founded because of my mother, surely I was different, more levelheaded. I told myself this while I shifted the camper into park in the lot of the university lofts near downtown, where we'd be staying for the week. It was June 4, and the place was empty for the summer.

"You'll enter through this gate over here," the loft director said, leading Nate and me through an opening in a tall security fence. "And your apartment is just on the other side of this courtyard."

We walked a short distance along the open grass in the direction that he had pointed. He used a ring of master keys to unlock the door of a meticulous apartment space that felt a bit like a hotel room without a TV. Two twin beds on opposite sides of the room were neatly made with crisp white sheets, and the tiles, counters, and kitchen all had the same even gray tone.

Nate looked inside the full-sized fridge and grinned. "Look, babe," he said, "it's a normal-sized fridge!"

I felt oddly embarrassed by his statement, like we were these deprived charity folk who didn't have access to common amenities while we begged our way across the country. I'd just as soon stay in the RV with its condensed fridge, hardly asking anybody for anything if I thought Nate was happy doing the same. I busied myself by moving—by setting my bag down on the bed and thanking the director.

"I'm thinking I can do tomorrow's miles on my own," I said to Nate after the director closed the door on his way out.

Nate was lying on his bed, his legs crossed, his hands propped behind his head.

"Really?" he asked. "How are you gonna get back?"

"Steve is meeting me with a group of runners," I said. "I could ask him to park at the finish and catch a ride to the start. That way, when we're done running the twelve miles, his car will be there, and he can give me a ride back. I thought it might be good for you to sleep in and just hang out."

"Really?" he said, sitting up, excited. "Is this part of your ploy so that I'll love Denver?"

I smiled. "Is it working?"

JUST VISITING

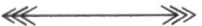

THE NEXT MORNING, SHORTLY after dawn, the sky glowed soft hues of blush and turquoise. I walked under the canopy of a cotton candy sky along the sleepy courtyard, cradling a cluster of keys from the apartment, car, and security gate in one hand, with my water bottle and a banana in the other. I pushed the gate open with my backside. It creaked a shrill sound into the quiet air, and I left.

Driving in the car to meet Steve's group, I took in the downtown buildings and empty sidewalks and felt a weight within my chest. I missed this place, or rather, the simplicity of being here with only myself to think about. There was a carelessness to my days then, one that I now understood I might never have again. Could I roll a joint for a day in the mountains? Could I take off on my own, buzzed on rounds of Prosecco, to pierce my nose? These were not things founders of nonprofits did, I noted.

Thirty minutes later, I arrived at the group meeting spot in the City of Golden. It was called Parfet Park, a quaint green space at the base of the mountains where I ended my run the day before.

"Ashley," Steve called out, pulling off his sports sunglasses and propping them on top of his white visor. He waved his hand once in the air.

"Steve," I called back, waving in return.

He stood with a group of eleven other runners under the shade of a maturing tree. Its leaves were vibrant and firm, just having bloomed for the summer. Underneath, a couple of the runners bounced in their sweat-wicking outfits. It was a cool morning with a hint of warmth to come. A dry, intense heat would ascend by high noon.

"Ashley, this is everybody," Steve said, introducing me.

I smiled and said hi as they introduced themselves one by one, knowing I wouldn't remember any of their names, wondering if it was obvious that I wouldn't, wondering if it was normal that I wouldn't and if it'd be okay if I asked their names later, or if doing that would make it seem like I wasn't listening to them now, like I wasn't because I was thinking about what was normal name-remembering etiquette. A woman in a teal tank top saved me from my thoughts.

"I can't believe you ran here from San Francisco," she said.

I shrugged, not knowing how to respond, not feeling fully comfortable in a group of strangers after three hundred hours of running alone. "It's true," I replied.

"I can almost vouch for her," Steve jumped in. "I've been auditing her miles since I met her on Tuesday."

"What?" I asked, amused. "Auditing my miles?"

"Yes," he replied. "To make sure you are really running across America."

I laughed at the thought. "Why wouldn't I *actually* be running across America?"

"I don't know." He shrugged. "People do odd things for attention."

I nodded at his point.

"But don't worry," he continued. "It appears you're actually doing it. You've run all the miles I've run with you, we're doing twelve miles as a group today, and I'll be joining you a few more times throughout Denver just to be sure."

"Sounds good to me," I said, unthreatened by the idea of someone tracking my miles.

"This is completely normal Steve behavior," a man offered. "He would audit miles."

The group nodded in agreement.

"If you'd really like to get back at him," another runner added, "try giving him a hug."

At that, the group laughed, and the whole exchange put me at ease. Steve was odd. The group was odd. I was odd. There was nothing to be anxious about, after all. I fit exactly into place as I always had with other runners—just another quirky person in a pair of running shoes.

Off in the run, everyone started to chat.

"I know a bit about MS," a woman said, running at my side after we'd departed from the park. "I'm a physical therapist, so I work with MS patients on their mobility." She was about my age and build—young and athletic, and she talked while running with ease. Conversation at our nine-thirty pace would be no problem at all for either of us.

"You do?" I asked. "That's great. There's such a big need to help MS patients with their movement, and not nearly enough attention and funding to support it."

"I agree," she replied. "I can make so much progress when I'm with a person. They move better. They feel better. They're more independent. But the second they don't meet their deductible or have coverage for their copay, that's it. They're gone. And all that progress we've made is lost."

"I know. It's frustrating," I said. "I got my degree in exercise and sports science, and just like anyone dedicated to exercise, there's a real motivation hurdle to overcome. With the disease on top of that, symptoms create more barriers that some can overcome. I'm not making excuses for people, but it is hard. The medication alone is astronomical."

"Is it?" she asked.

"It is. Thousands of dollars per month," I replied. "My dad's worked really hard to take care of my family and my mom's medical treatments. Plus, he's my mom's main caregiver, so when it comes to ways they could spend more money—maybe on a housekeeper or part-time aid, it's hard to imagine there'd be extra for PT."

"Ugh. I never really thought about all of the other expenses," she said.

"Yeah."

I didn't know what else to add. There was so much more—the never-ending financial pressure, my father drinking to manage the stress, their house piled high with garbage, and me traveling around the world to avoid it until now. What could be accomplished by sharing more of the truth? I changed the subject.

"I used to live here for a bit, up in Boulder," I said. "I was on track for PT myself. Got accepted into Regis."

"Really? What happened?"

"I got offered a job on a cruise ship," I said, smiling. "So I decided to do that instead."

"A cruise ship? Now that sounds cool," she said. "What'd you do for work?"

Our conversation took the positive turn I was hoping for. She was pulled into the fascination of my past work, and, in turn, I learned about her as well. Her name was Kara, and she was a single, young professional in Denver. She loved to run and live near the mountains. After this, she'd meet up with her friends at Washington Park for an afternoon of canned beer and grass volleyball. Come Monday, she'd get dressed in her dark slacks and polyester-blend button-up top and go to work, where she'd assess the mobility range of an empty-nester with a new knee replacement, writing down the flexion range on her progress report paper and then taking them through a series of tests and advancing exercises. I knew it well. It was exactly the life I had imagined for myself before I boarded the cruise ship, before all of this.

I learned these things about Kara while we ran along the Cherry Creek bike path, a paved two-lane track with a dashed line painted up the center, one of many in the metro Denver area. It looked like the highways I had been running, only narrower and void of the occasional semi-truck whooshing past and blowing off my visor.

The fastest vehicles were the bicycles that'd approach every so often with an "On your left!" shout from the rider. Our group of twelve would shift, the bicycle would pass, and then we'd fan back out. We did this without breaking stride—our bobbing heads bouncing up and down like pistons, moving together, then out, running two by two.

My mother had moved like this as well. Not as a runner, but a horse rider, up and down on her pinto horse named Goat Cheese. She'd run her hand down the length of her horse's glossy coat, her fingers feeling every fiber of hair beneath them. She'd find the firm, leather saddle, then lift her booted foot into the stirrup and hoist her petite and mighty frame onto the horse's back. She'd lean forward and stroke the mane. One controlled kick with her heel, and Goat Cheese moved into stride.

The Wisconsin fields were honey colored, like her long, blonde hair, and she heard only her breathing and the gallop of hooves against dry ground. The warm summer air brushed across her skin. The rhythm of the animal's body beneath her danced with the movement of her own. It was joy. It was freedom. In her mind, it remained.

"I had my body back," my mom said to me one morning, the look of peacefulness on her face hard to explain. "The dream was so vivid I thought it was real."

I didn't speak. I sat gently on the edge of her bed, cautious that I'd frighten this lucid moment away—her recalling a dream, her actually being able to articulate it to me.

"I was riding on my horse." She smiled. "Jesus was there. He said I'd be healthy again, in heaven."

She was silent for a moment.

"It was perfect," she said. And at that, finally, she let the tears come.

I grew in deep admiration of her the more I learned about her and what the symptoms of MS had taken. This run wasn't just an athletic achievement for me. I was proud of her. Made immobile for days, dependent, stripped of the parts she once claimed as identity, a graceful horse rider, slalom water-skier, pianist, singer. The disease raged, and still, she glowed. Others would benefit from knowing this too, knowing her, knowing who she was.

Still, the endeavor hadn't been easy. The motorhome had broken down multiple times, costing thousands of dollars and delaying days of progress. Spade made me into a fool twice—once when I gave him the credit card number and again when I didn't kick his ass to the curb the second I found out. And the mornings had become a routine of Nate wanting to sleep in and me nagging him to get out of bed so I could run.

All that work, and I had only raised $19,130.53 so far.

Mostly, it was less glamorous than what people thought, and all I could do was smile and nod when others asked in wonder about my life. I couldn't tell them about what was hard because I hadn't learned how to fix it yet. The only thing I knew I was doing well was the running, and even that I'd be done with for the next four days.

Once again, Denver presented itself as the most delightful escape.

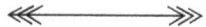

"YOU'RE A LITTLE DIFFERENT," my friend Emily said to me later that day.

"Different how?" I asked, furrowing my brow.

She and I shared a plaid blanket that evening at Denver's long-standing summer community event, Jazz in the Park. She was Steph's roommate in college and now a full-time resident of Denver, Colorado. Days prior, Emily knew I was coming through town and invited me to meet her at City Park for drinks and live music. I accepted, and Nate took off to play "footy" with the group of Australians he'd found on Facebook.

"I'm not sure. Maybe... more serious?" she said in a question. She turned her knees from the stage toward me.

"I'm not serious. You're drunk," I joked. Wanting to be fun and relax, I reclined on my elbows, watching a saxophonist jive out a soft, solo melody. Emily poured me a second heaping cup of wine.

"I'm not drunk," she replied. "Just a little buzzed."

I smiled. "Me too."

"It's not a bad thing," she said. "It's cool what you're doing. And it also seems like a lot of responsibility."

"Maybe," I said, lying myself flat. We sat on the blanket under the canopy of an oak tree. A disco ball was strung from the branches above. I watched it spin and twinkle, feeling my lips go numb. "Right now, it's just a lot of running."

We sat together, not talking for a few moments, listening to the melody.

"What are you going to do with all the money?" she asked.

"What do you mean?" I replied, sitting up. "I'm going to give it away."

"Aren't you worried, though? About doing all this work and not having any of it for yourself when you're done?"

Her questions reminded me of Nate's. Lately, there were fewer conversations about enjoying the journey, and more about what we'd do when we got home. I didn't have a good answer. I had a growing sense that I had only just begun.

I took a deep breath and tipped a gulp of wine into my mouth. "I'm not worried," I replied, "I'm enjoying this. I'll figure out home when I get there."

The musician swayed, closing their eyes. I watched and thought of my mother. Did it matter how far ahead I planned? What's to come would come either way.

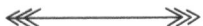

THE NEXT MORNING, I shook off my hangover with a 3.2-mile hike up the Sanitas trail in Boulder with an old coworker while Nate slept in.

Marching up the single-track dirt trail under a warm morning sun, smelling subtly of stale alcohol, sweat beaded on my brow. My head throbbed, but my legs were steady and strong. To get here, I drove the car north out of Denver on I-70, as I had done a number of times in my past. The road slanted up until it crested the ridge that overlooked the valley of Boulder, Colorado—a free-spirited town at the base of five rock formations at the edge of the Rocky Mountains, the Flatirons. The car crested the overlook, and I, hazy and slow, knew that the grandeur of being here far outweighed staying in bed.

Hiking up the trail with Amber at my back, I turned my head to ask, "Did you bring green?"

She snorted from behind. "Did I bring green?"

Looking forward again, I kept moving. "Perfect."

We reached a high clearing twenty minutes later and took a seat on a rounded slab of rock. Next to me, Amber took off her day pack and zipped open the front compartment. There, tucked neatly into a mesh pocket, was a joint. She took out a lighter and flicked it. Back in the day, we'd roll the joint together and then light up in her car before our waitressing shifts. If there were time, we'd float to the grocery store next to our work for to-go sushi.

Smoking with her now, Amber and I sat upon one of the Flatirons' five crests, which jutted out from the rugged and forested earth below. I remember looking upon these five faces from my

North Boulder apartment one February morning, just weeks after I'd arrived here for the first time. The rocks were smooth and tilted toward the heavens, snow-covered and glowing orange. I stared, feeling like the luckiest girl in the world. Every week, I spent hours by myself in these woods, working my way up the hardened, worn trail to the rocks—up, over, and through them—then back down again to my Jetta parked in the trailhead lot.

The City of Boulder spread out to the east in front of us in full view, where the land opened up level and wide in the direction that I was headed. Boulder's three reservoirs reflected the pale blue sky up from the ground like mirrors on the land. Tall trees shadowed the pockets of homes underneath, and trails here were as plentiful as the roads. It was just as dazzling as I remembered. Maybe more.

"I love it here," I confessed, feeling nostalgic.

She stared as well, nodding in agreement. "It's pretty great."

The morning drifted away, and before long, I was back in Denver with Nate. We'd meet up with his Aussie friends, drink beer, play footy. We'd sleep, go to hot yoga, drink Bloody Marys. We'd ride bikes around downtown, stroll a chalk festival, listen to bongo drummers. We'd walk side by side, hold hands, flirt. He'd look at me. I'd smile back. We'd talk—about living here, paid work, buying a home, starting roots. I was enamored again by him, by a backyard of mountains, by the steadiness of being in one place.

If it hadn't been for David, I may have ignored all the reasons I needed to leave.

CHAPTER FIFTEEN
Running Home

"**THIS DISEASE HAS TAKEN** most of my hearing, and some days it takes my running. But with people like Ashley fighting for a cure, it will never take my hope."

David stood next to me on stage with a microphone in his hand. Tears welled in his eyes, then streamed down his face. The audience of more than a hundred supporters sat silently on their metal folding chairs, sobered by David's harsh reality. Many were his friends who saw him every week at the pub's Wednesday night running club. They'd meet, run three miles around Cheesman Park, and then convene back at the pub for beers and pasta. David was a group leader. Some of them never knew he lived with MS.

Hours prior, Nate and I arrived at the Irish Snug restaurant and descended the stairs into a bevy of new and old faces. I stepped into the crowd to talk about the run, my mother, and the disease, and Nate joined our friends to help with raffle sales and drinks.

That I spent the last three days drinking and smoking weed had little effect on my internal compass to do this work. I wasn't faking one thing and doing another. I was both. I had jumped into this charity and shed myself of these habits like an old coat, or so I thought. I ran and fundraised and advocated, and as I went, I found that I was still the girl who relished a good joint on the beach.

It was just that I was also now a girl running across America, wanting to raise half a million dollars for MS. Some of these things were more important than others. This, I knew. Still, like well-loved clothing I had grown out of, there were times when I found myself wanting to try on my old ways, to remember what it was like, to see how it fit.

By the time I stood next to David on stage, tearing up with the rest of them while he shared his MS story, my throat was raw from telling my own story throughout the night. I talked about my mother and the strength of her character. I talked about my run and why I was on the road for five hours each day.

At David's side, I held back a sob and remembered why I had to leave—that this run was bigger than me. That we all needed something to hope for.

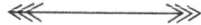

MY MOTHER'S HOPE, THOUGH, was not on my running or for a cure. It was in Jesus. He walked this earth thousands of years ago and guaranteed her and everyone else a place in heaven if they just believed. And she did, more than most, I can say. It's why she accepted her struggles, she told me. Why she smiled so, come what may.

"Ashley, tell them." She had nudged at my side after I spoke at a Lions Club luncheon before I left for San Francisco.

"Tell them what, Mom?" I whispered back. The aged men in their business suits stabbed their salads with metal forks and leaned into each other in conversation, hovering over black coffee in porcelain cups.

"About why MS doesn't scare me," she said. "Tell 'em about Jesus."

Straightening myself, I would do no such thing. I shooed at her, embarrassed that she'd use my run as an evangelist opportunity.

I couldn't reconcile her God and the one I knew, who met me somewhere else altogether—beyond the stained glass windows and hymnal singing. God moved in the wind, in the birds, in me, upon a ship where I wondered about doing this run in the first place. God met me here, on the road, in this charity—a discovery that still felt too personal to speak about. Because, if I was being honest with myself, when it came to my mother—God and I—we had some sorting out to do.

If I could name it, it would be anger. A youthful "fuck you" that led me to do what I wanted—binge drink, casual sex, occasional drug use. If what my mother got is what one gets, then what was the point?

And then, simply, God gave me a point. A reason to run farther. And the more I ran, the less angry I felt.

By the time I left Denver on an ominous, gray morning, I felt no anger at all. I felt buoyant and happy, a curious notion to me as I was leaving my beloved snowcapped mountains behind—the place I yearned for and planned to return to, the place I thought about arriving at when I thought about how desperately I wanted to arrive somewhere.

Yet, beyond them now, I remained lively. Maybe more so. Just as well, I thought to myself of the mountains at my back as I ran down a wet and well-traveled highway, their view obscured by a sheet of overcast clouds. I was running on my line again, the white paint that colored the paved path before me, with twenty-four miles to tick away. No need to linger where I should not stay.

What pulled at me was ahead, farther east.

It was home. I was running home.

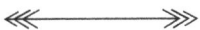

"**SO YOU BETTER RUN.** Run fast for your mother, fast for your father," I sang aloud, Florence and the Machine thumping through my earbuds. "Run for your children, for your sisters and brothers. Leave all your love 'n' your longing behind. Can't carry it with you if you want to survive. The dog days are o-va-ah, the dog days are goooone. Can you hear the horses-say-yay-yas, cuz heeeeere... they... coooome?"

I sang and ran, ran and sang, moving east along Highway 34 when I crossed my fourth state line into Nebraska on a beautiful

June day. This was The Good Life, the bullet-riddled highway sign said, a cowboy waving his hat in the air upon a bucking stallion. To my left and right, fields of vibrant reeds stretched out in every direction, swaying in a gentle breeze to my shouting. Wildflowers painted the highway with natural shades of cream and honey. The sky was the perfect touch of clear and bright. Full summer was in bloom now, and I was in the Midwest, made evident to me by the keen sense of familiarity that flooded my senses in the four days since I'd run out of Denver.

"That's the exit where the hobo thought I was stopping to give him a ride," I'd say to Nate as we moved along. Or, "I stayed in that hotel right over there."

I had been along these roads before, during the sixteen-hour driving sessions stretched between home and Colorado. Once, I had even imagined what it would be like to run the distance between the two states—that I would mail supplies to UPS along the way, that I would run to my supplies and sleep in hotels for the summer. It was a thought that had been forgotten, faded from my consciousness as just a whim until I actually started doing it—running from Colorado to Wisconsin, and the memory of thinking such a thing resurfaced.

I chuckled at the lost epiphany, then recalled it in conversation with Lauren, the high school cross-country runner who opted to sit at my side at the Brush City swimming pool after running six miles with me that morning. Her teammates swam nearby—chasing each other and splashing in the cool water at the bottom of a thirty-foot slide.

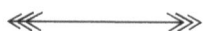

"SO YOU ALWAYS WANTED to do this then?" she asked of my memory.

I shook my head no. "I didn't," I replied, kicking my feet back and forth in the pool. My ankles shone bright against bronze legs. "I got my degree in exercise and sports science. I thought I was going to be a physical therapist."

"Why'd you change your mind?" she asked, moving a long dreadlock from her face, plastic beads dangled from the ends.

"Something better came up," I said, looking at Nate on the other side of the pool, resting on a deck chair with his arm draped across his face. A group of children in the water screeched in delight. The rough concrete pressed into the back of my legs, and I thought of walking to retrieve my towel that lay at Nate's side, but decided rather to stay where I was.

"I got offered a job on a cruise ship, so I chose to travel the world instead. Then I left that to do this, so here I am."

By this time, it was late afternoon, and the sun was hot. I dipped myself underwater for a refresher, then pulled myself back onto the deck next to the girl. She was in her third year at the high school. Her coach had heard about my run and rallied up his team of teenagers to escort me through the area. They had arrived at the Camry that morning and did what high school cross-country runners do—they ran and chattered and buzzed with energy and laughed without breaking stride.

Being with them reminded me of my own high school cross-country experience—a place where I felt accepted, an individual among a group of others, while I wrestled with the uncertainty of being a teenager in a new school when my mother's health was declining. I wondered how Lauren fit in among her peers and why she sat next to me now instead of being with them—if she felt as out of place as I had at her age and if she steeled herself inside to be strong about being alone.

"Will you go back to cruise ships after you finish in New York?" she asked, breaking my thoughts.

"Probably not," I said. "I think I'm going to do something with the charity."

"Really?" she asked. "Like what?"

"Something like this," I said, shifting on my legs. "Help people run across America for MS."

She turned her face from the water and looked at me. "Maybe someday I could?" she asked.

I returned her gaze and smiled, "You can if you want to."

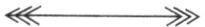

AFTER WE LEFT THE pool, Nate and I drove to a place in town to pick up the tow dolly he had pushed for. Purchasing it was a decision to make moving camp every three days more convenient.

"The tow connects here," the shop owner said with a grunt, picking up the front of the dolly with some effort and steering its ball to the hitch before slamming it in place with a bang.

"And you put these two ramps in the notches here," he continued, bending down to retrieve each ramp from the dirt, one at a time, and placing them so. "Then you drive the car up until the wheel hits this bar here."

The ramps were grated and heavy. The tires of the car were intended to sit in a low steel bowl and then be tethered to the platform with basket straps.

"These are webbed nylon with a working load max of ten thousand pounds," the man said, holding a mass of green straps in his gloved hand, each six feet in length. A flat, steel hook held the strap in place at the front, then the nylon basket lay over the top of the wheel and was ratcheted into place in the back.

"They won't move or shake, even in the rain," he concluded.

I nodded like I knew exactly what he was talking about, like I had thought all along about nylon straps moving or shaking in the rain.

To get the car off the dolly, first, the ramps had to come off the tow. They tucked into each other just under the front bumper of the car and tightened into place with a long, L-shaped screw. Once the ramps were in place below the wheels, I'd squeezed the ratchet and worked to pop it straight, releasing the basket straps. Dirt and grime from the road clung to the straps, which billowed when the straps were released and pulled off each wheel. Then the car could be reversed down the ramps, and all the dolly pieces tucked back into place.

I would do all this on my own for the first time without gloves, a day later. Turning the L-screw, my hand scraped across the top of the steel ramp like a cheese grater, bloodying my knuckles and causing me to shout.

"Fuck!"

Nate ran from the side of the motorhome where he worked to connect the water. "What? What, babe? Are you okay?"

"Stupid. Fucking. Thing," I said, dancing in pain, pressing hard on my mangled hand, applying pressure.

"What? Let me see," he said, coming to my side.

"No," I groaned. " Fuck. Just let me be for a minute." The pain throbbed up my arm. There was nothing to be done that I couldn't do myself.

After dinner, he went out on his own. The next morning, I found a new pair of deer skin gloves on the counter.

"These are nice," I said, holding them. Their leather was smooth and strong, the perfect barrier between my hand and the dirty dolly job.

"Yeah, I figured we only need to learn that lesson once, right?" he said with a smile.

"Right."

I tossed the gloves down on the dinette table and picked up my bowl of oatmeal, peanut butter, and craisins.

"May have to go out later than normal tonight," I said. "The heat's really not letting up until after dinner."

"Yeah, okay, babe," Nate agreed. "Let's give it a try."

Looking outside the window in the thick summer air, the sky began to lighten with sunrise. It was early, but it'd be hot soon enough. I pulled on a pair of socks, tied on my running shoes, and walked out the door.

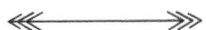

ON THE HIGHWAY RUNNING, I heard only the sloshing of the water in my new hydration backpack, the crunching of gravel underfoot, and my breath moving in and out. It was rhythmic and steady, a constant—the trusted melody to my life. The vibrant fields, too, remained. They spanned out in front of me until they met the sky, a dome of color that reached far above me and behind.

As a car approached, I'd raise my hand each time, waving. The driver, too, was already waving back.

I ran and felt a richness of comfort in these surroundings, as if I were already home. I ticked off my morning miles with ease, one by one, within this coziness.

Nate stood at the car, sweating through his tank top, when I arrived for one last dose of electrolytes.

"Looking good, babe. You're crushing these miles."

"Thanks," I replied, chipper. I popped the plastic top off a water jug and poured. "Feels good out here, like I know where I'm going. Plus"—I took a bite of the banana he offered—"I'm running down."

Nearing the town of Cambridge, elevation 2,264, I had dropped three thousand feet since leaving Denver eleven days prior. Just then, a car slowed down, pulled over, and came to a stop directly in front of the Camry. A woman emerged from the driver's seat.

"Hi there." The woman waved, walking toward us.

"Hi," Nate and I replied in unison.

"My name is Lorette," she said, extending her hand. She shook Nate's first, then mine. "I'm a writer for the *Valley Voice*, just up the way in Cambridge," she said, gesturing toward the highway with her compact, spiral-bound notebook. "A local gave me a ring. Said he came across you on his bike earlier. Said you're running across America for your mother?"

"Yeah, that's right," I replied, recalling the biker who'd coasted at my side for a few minutes after sunrise. He had come across the car, parked and waiting for me, which had been wrapped in vinyl advertising in Denver to match the RV.

"It's just a local paper. Nothing big, ya know. But I'd love to do a story on you if that's okay?"

Lorette couldn't have been much older than me. A crown of glossy dark hair topped her head, and the skin on her face was too bright and young to hold the lines that appeared when she talked.

"It's farm country out here, ya know. But these are good people who'd love to read about what you're doing. Shouldn't take but a minute."

"You don't have to ask me twice." I smiled. "I'd love to tell you about my run."

"Great," she said, tucking her hair behind her ear and flipping open the notebook. She clicked the top of her pen. "So, tell me how long you've been running?"

"I started March 22 at the Golden Gate Bridge. So what is that? What's the date?"

Lorette looked at her watch. "June 22."

"Oh my gosh. Yay!" I said, too giddy for such a silly coincidence. "Three months to the date!"

"So you've been running for three months already?"

"Yup."

"How much longer do you have to go?"

I tipped my palm up and down in an estimate gesture. "Eh, about another three months. I'm scheduled to finish in New York near the end of September."

She scribbled on the pad and then flipped to a new sheet. "Are you worried at all about keeping that timeline?"

"Nope."

"Why not? Do you have any injuries? Are you sore?"

I shook my head no. "Do two blisters count as injuries?"

"That's all that's happened to you? Just two blisters? No other injuries?" She looked at me with eyes wide, then at Nate, then back at me. "How many miles is that?"

"Right around sixteen hundred. I'm about halfway."

"You've run sixteen hundred miles in three months, and you're fine?" she said, her mouth agape. "How is that possible?"

Fortunately, I had been given 347 hours on the road to consider her question. It was more than being physically capable of running it, of which I had been well equipped. It was the example I'd been given in my youth, strength in the face of adversity when my family was rocked, yet again, by persistent MS attacks. It was the rooting I had in wellness despite some of my destructive habits. It was the hours I spent studying exercise science, not knowing how I'd use that vital knowledge now. It was winning a debate in class, voted as the top presenter by my peers long before I'd started my own charity. It was the model of faith given to me to trust what I knew to be true long before I could prove its existence. It was accepting the death of one plan for another, the beginning with what little I had, the showing up when practicality would suggest otherwise. It was none of these things alone, but all of them together. The pieces of my life fitting into place.

I told her this, the string of my life, as simply as I could—with a shrug and a sentence, because how else could I explain it? "It's what I've been made to do."

Back at the camper, Lorette followed us inside. We reconvened there as the discussion continued, and I grew hungry.

"You really don't mind that I look around?" she asked. "I don't need to be here if you're busy."

"I don't mind if you don't mind that I eat," I replied. "It's a neat little space—if you don't mind blue. It's been lent to us by a family back home." I opened the fridge and started to rummage around. She studied the postcards and bumper stickers we stuck to the wall.

"America's Loneliest Highway?" she asked, pointing to the card we bought in Austin, Nevada, just after we crossed paths with Brains On Bikes. Nate and I checked in on Anne and Gundy often. They were nearing the last leg of their journey. In seventeen days, they'd be finished with their ride.

"That's in Nevada," I said, holding a bag of salt-and-vinegar chips in my hand, shaking them into a heaping pile on my plate. I used the plate only because Lorette was there. Otherwise, I'd eat straight from the bag like an animal.

"And is it lonely?" Lorette asked, leaning in closer to view the desolate highway pictured on the card.

"I liked it," I said.

"It was lonely," Nate countered.

Lorette laughed at our banter. As it happens, she was young—a farm girl from Nebraska who had just graduated with a degree in communication from the University of Nebraska, Kearney. "I thought I'd move away somewhere," she said, talking of her post-college plan. "But then a job opened up here in Cambridge, and I don't know." She shrugged. "It's nice to be close to family."

Like me, she was a middle child. But unlike me, both of her parents were healthy. Her father was a farmer, and her mother worked for the city council.

I gave her the good parts of mine, as I did—a shallow version of a truth too harsh. What she heard was that my mom was doing okay. That she lived with disability and poor fine motor skills, but that we were fortunate that she had a great outlook and my father as her full-time caregiver. That they gathered up savings to purchase rental units so my dad could spend his days taking care of her. That, in spite of it all, they were set on giving us kids a normal childhood where I got to play sports and they never missed a game; where we took family trips to Disney World and had regular movie nights; that I had always been supported—through college and years thereafter; that my parents funded the charity's inception.

What I left out were the things that truly mattered when it came to the disease—which were the same things that invoked a look of pity that I simply could not shoulder. That my father drank too much to manage the stress and depression; that my mother drank too because there was hardly anything else to do when one was mostly confined to the couch; that the house was a mess—piled high with garbage and emotions that wouldn't be sorted out in any certain amount of time; that even though they appeared well-off, they were one long hospital stay away from losing it all; that this is why I ran—that we were a charity case, after all.

She'd never hear this from me or my family. They were the heavy, intimate things our pride would never let us say.

That night, after dinner, I ran. I laced up my Asics as the temperature dropped from a jarring 85.2 degrees to 81, to 78, to 74, to 68.

Thick air receded.

Crickets chirped.

Darkness ushered me in.

"Are you sure you don't want me to tail you?" Nate asked.

"I'll be okay," I replied.

I tucked my phone into the chest pocket of my pack and grabbed a neon reflective vest from the pocket in the door. The car's overhead light beamed its artificial glow like a spotlight into the cab.

"My eyes'll adjust to the darkness, and I'll turn on the flashlight if I see a car." I wanted to reassure him of my safety and that

I could manage on my own. Not like in Nevada, when I went out for an evening run and he insisted on coasting at my back for an hour, the hazard lights tick-clicking the entire time, which was no way to enjoy a run, I told him. He needed to ensure my safety, he told me. I had been fine for all the years before we met, I said back.

And now he was beginning to trust my senses, dropping me off on the side of the road in Nebraska in the full of night. That or he just couldn't be bothered to challenge me anymore.

Blanketed in darkness on Highway 34, after the brake lights of the Camry disappeared, I *was* okay, as I had said, but still, adrenaline coursed. I was out there. *Out-there* out there, miles from any sizable city that'd shine streetlights into the evening sky, and because of it, I was within a depth of black that I had rarely encountered.

And yet, even in the inky black night, the landscape revealed itself.

The road lines shone ashen pale against charcoal, like stones upon a trail. The grass met the road at the gravel shoulder, then sloped abruptly into a ditch. Beyond that, a wooden post fence linked together with scrawny lengths of wire.

Walking along at first, I felt a heightened sense of my surroundings. Gravel crunched louder than at day beneath my sneakers, prickling my ears. The texture of summer air enveloped my nostrils—damp, sweet, grassy. And I was more aware of my body—where my pack touched the tops of my shoulders, the elastic band of my shorts wrapped around my waist, the bottoms of my feet in a cushy pair of cotton socks.

Moving into stride, it wasn't long before the night's wonders appeared.

First came the stars, a thousand million hundred billion of them; bitty bright flecks of twinkle on the bubble of space above me—more than I recalled seeing before or ever cared to think about. Had there always been this many stars?

I ran and looked up.

Amazed, I looked around, looked behind me, turned around and ran backward, looked up and turned forward. I stretched my arms out and turned.

Surely, I looked ridiculous, looking up, running, and turning about in circles. But I was alone. Fully alone. More alone than I was at any other time, with Nate or running this path during the day. Even with the confidence to fully be myself around others, there were parts of me that I'd hide, like this, unabashed joy like a child turning about in the night. A tiny ripple of laughter at this freedom jumped from my lips. Yes, I was just fine on my own.

Sometime later, the stars descended to the earth in equal number, sparkling on my plane in the vast open fields—little flashes of light. If I hadn't known better, I'd have thought I was hallucinating that the stars *had* descended and that I could touch them. But I did know better. These glittering lights were fireflies—a winged, soft-bodied beetle with luminescent organs that flourished throughout the summer months across the Midwest. As a child, I had chased them throughout the yard, trapped them inside of mason jars, and pressed the jar up to my nose, spellbound by their glow.

They floated above the grasses now, dancing upon the air, ablaze.

If I could liken what I've learned of MS to that which I now know, it would be this: like running into the night.

"In time, we decided to live the life we wanted," my father recalled of their early years after my mom's diagnosis. After two years of being carted around by my grandmother to every neurological specialist within an hour's drive, my parents had had enough. It was, after all the tests and retests, MS. They would step into it.

The most daunting aspect of the disease is the unknown. There is no telling what will or wouldn't become. She could need a wheelchair, or she may be fine. It could take decades, or it could happen in a year. It could be her eyes, her ears, her throat—any voluntary part of her body that was controlled by the nervous system. The only way to know was to wake up and assess what was still there.

And with a heightened sense of how the disease had changed her life, my mother stepped into the darkness and found that the Jill she had always known was still there, with plenty left to experience beyond the life she'd once lived. Even that there were surprising beauties to be found here too.

"It's been a blessing," my mother said of her MS. It was a test of her faith and a reason to drop the charade of pretending to be anything she wasn't for the comfort of others. The insignificant details of her life prior to diagnosis disappeared within this new setting, and she found that, actually, she never needed those superficial things in the first place. Even within the darkness, she found beauty because her power was not bound to her circumstances but rather in her perception of them.

In the days that followed this evening run, beauty came to me like the fireflies had that night–abundant, illuminating.

"I picked these for you," a little girl said, standing on the side of the highway, holding out a small bushel of seeded morsels. I bit into one, and bursts of strawberry gushed into my mouth. A tidal wave of sweetness rushed through my blood. Had strawberries always been this good? I closed my eyes and, for a moment, felt only the delicious, tender fruit between my lips, like a downpour of rain upon desert land.

"Wow," I moaned. "These. Are. Amazing!"

The girl was a farmer's daughter, and she ran from the front stoop at her home near Cambridge down her dirt drive to greet me as I ran past. Lorette had published her story about me in the local paper, and now everyone knew the solo woman running along Highway 34 was the one running across America for her mother.

This girl's father had slowed next to me while biking past an hour earlier. Upon arriving home, he told his daughter that the woman from the paper running across America would be by the house soon. The girl pulled on her tiny rubber boots and gathered up what she had to give, then met me with an eager hand waving through the air. She embodied what I would come to learn of Nebraskans–they'd gather up what they had to give and meet me with an eager hand.

From Cambridge, I ran through the quiet towns of Arapahoe, Holdredge, and Minden–past giant silos and working mills, past worn churches and frequented bars. I ran twenty-three miles, twenty-five miles, twenty-eight miles until midnight again to avoid the scorching sun. I'd rip off my shoes and place my feet on ice packs. I'd lie across the motorhome floor in the cooled air, AC blasting, with a damp wash cloth across my pulsing face. We'd park in vacant lots, and people came by just to say hi. A friend's mother drove an hour one way just to visit. She picked up our laundry, washed it, folded it, and returned it along with a four-course meal. Groups of runners were notified. They showed up. We ran.

CHAPTER SIXTEEN
The Good Life

I WAS LYING ON the bed under a soft fleece blanket late into the morning—after running seventeen miles, after I inhaled a foot-long chicken sandwich, a bag of chips, and three cookies from the Subway shop in town—when my father called.

I was thoroughly drained by my usual morning activities in a way I hadn't experienced yet. The summer heat was a constant now, and it hollowed me out of both nutrition and energy. I set my morning alarm earlier and earlier, but the reprieve of doing so was fractional. The sun would rise, and with it, the temperature. Even before it rose, its blaze was present—a torrid radiating furnace waiting to crest the horizon. I could endure it, but still, it wore on me.

Nothing that can't be fixed with a nap and an ice-cold Coca-Cola, I reminded myself, pulling the covers to my chin in the air-conditioned motorhome. I was always just one sleep and a sugar rush away from another good run.

"Hey, Dad," I said through the phone, my voice giving away my state—fatigued and still.

"Hey, kiddo, were you sleeping?"

"Getting there," I told him. "I just laid down. What's up?"

"Ah, just calling to finalize plans for our visit, that's all. It can wait. Want to call me back later?" he asked.

"Yeah. If you don't mind? Call you back in a few hours?"

"You bet, kiddo."

We hung up, and I clicked through my phone to silence the ringer. I opened my Facebook app and updated my status, typing in: "Tired doesn't even cover it." Then I set my phone down and fell into an abyss of deep sleep.

Sleep, of course, just like eating, hydrating, and avoiding extreme temperatures, was a critical piece to my success thus far. My body was my vehicle, and to keep it running, I came prepared.

"The hormones released when you sleep are necessary for muscle recovery, mental clarity, and overall performance," my exercise physiology professor stated to the lecture hall full of students. "Growth hormone for repair, leptin for appetite control, prolactin for immune support. All these hormones and more are released when you sleep. The more sleep you get, the better your results."

I had always been a good sleeper, and my high school cross-country coach harped on us to get eight hours of it each night, but now I was experiencing *why* that was so important. Back then, I had been focused on results for my future physical therapy clients. Now, I became my own subject.

Just that morning, a marathoner from Lincoln ran by my side, asking me about such things.

"How many times have you hit the wall?" he questioned.

We were moving through a sizable Nebraskan town called Hastings. We ran past a McDonald's, an auto sales center, and a fun little roadhouse restaurant named Kitty's—where I noted to come back later for a burger, but ended up wanting a quick Subway meal instead because that was an option too.

"I haven't," I replied. Another semi-truck filled with corn feed passed us from behind, moving east, as we were, along Highway 6. "I split the miles each day into two—a chunk in the morning like we're doing now, and then I'll do what's left in the afternoon after lunch and a nap."

The thing he had asked about, the wall, was a common experience for endurance athletes—a sudden and rapid loss of energy resulting in extreme fatigue, muscle soreness, and mental breakdown. It was so widespread and challenging during endurance events that one could identify those who were experiencing it and those who weren't. It was a drooping of the shoulders, a shuffling of the feet, a downcast, sunken look in the eyes. It had a haunting name and could be so overwhelming that some would drop from races to end it rather than endure it.

The condition, I knew, could be explained.

"There are three metabolic pathways for the body during exercise," my college professor continued. "Phosphagen, glycolic, and oxidative. Food is converted into ATP, which is stored in limited amounts within your muscles." He underlined *limited amounts* on the whiteboard. "Once ATP is depleted, so is the *power*."

By now, I had lost the eight pounds I purposely gained before I started in California—stored fat for energy reserves. Somewhere between the west side of the Rockies and now, I had become the lean version of myself I was accustomed to from my years as an athlete. Skin on my upper arm pulled tight around my shoulder, veins visible up my calves, pulsing with deoxygenated blood, and six neat squares of muscle rippled across my midsection. I ate whatever I wanted, as much as I wanted, and still, I leaned out. I hoped it would be enough to get me to New York.

The body eventually runs out of reserves, both stored ATP and extra fat, and unless an athlete fuels properly during exercise, they experience the loss of power my professor taught about—sprinting becomes a run, becomes a jog, becomes a slog as the body moves from one main metabolic system to the next until there's nothing left to metabolize except the slow and painful conversion of muscle into energy like I had experienced myself during my first impromptu marathon.

Running like that without fuel on repeat across the country wouldn't just mean a plethora of painful runs. It meant nagging, chronic injuries. It meant the toxic breakdown of muscle tissue. Instead, I was splitting the distance in two runs—eating before, during, and after each run, and also napping most afternoons. Doing this, I wasn't just trying to avoid a difficult wall experience. I was trying to stay out of the hospital.

I awoke an hour or so later to the stillness of a slumbering motorhome. Nate had dozed off on the couch as well. A book, split at the spine, was open across his chest. I sat up slowly and placed my feet gently on the worn carpet. I tiptoed to the bathroom, peed a small amount of dark urine that told me I was in need of electrolytes, and then flushed the toilet by standing on the plastic step that opened the chute to the holding tank below. The sound of the forced water swishing into the bowl is what woke Nate. Everything had a noise.

"Hey there," I said, coming from the bathroom and taking a seat on the dinette bench.

"Hey." He stretched, groggy. "What time is it?"

"Just before one," I replied. "We've got some time, but we should probably go grocery shopping this afternoon."

The days had begun to stretch out. The sun was up before 6:00 a.m. and not setting until after 8:00 p.m. I awoke and ran. Then we'd wait the length of the day—eating, napping, running errands, poking around town looking at whatever there was to look at—sometimes something, oftentimes nothing—before we'd go back out so I could finish for the day. We had all the time in the world, with nowhere else to be and not much else to do.

"All right." He agreed, still lying across the length of the couch. "What'd your dad have to say?"

"I've gotta call him back. He just wants to talk about plans for their visit."

"You still want them to get a hotel?" He sat up.

"I think it makes sense for both my mom and us, but they're fully booked in Lincoln because of the holiday, so are you okay if they stay here?"

In just forty-eight hours, my parents and younger sister, Dawn, would drive 558 miles from Brookfield, Wisconsin, to us in Lincoln, Nebraska, to spend the Fourth of July holiday with Nate and me in the motorhome. I was giddy with anticipation. It'd be the first time we'd seen each other since I left home in March, since Nate proposed in Tahoe, since I'd run halfway across the country.

As he and I talked, I unconsciously played with a four-stone amethyst ring on my left ring finger. It was a gift he'd bought me on the cruise ship after I thought to run across America, but before I actually left to do it. He wanted me to have something special from him before I left, and he was always into buying nice things. He placed a black velvet box in my hands and showed me the ring that went on my right hand. Then, after the ringless proposal in Tahoe, we switched it to the left—as a placeholder, he promised. Now, we discussed him sharing a thirty-foot motorhome with half my family.

"It'll be fine, babe. Just have 'em bring a tent. Your mum and dad can have the bed, Dawn on the couch, and us in the tent outside."

I gave him a look. "You've never been tent camping before."

"I've done this with you," he said playfully about our van life adventure. "It can't be much different."

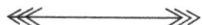

AS HE FOUND, TWO nights later, when he and I lay side by side on the ground under the canopy of my family's four-person nylon tent, it *was* different. The tent was army green—the same color as my father's Chevy Malibu, which had rolled up the campground's gravel drive a touch after 2:00 p.m., just as my father had planned.

They had risen before the sun, filled their to-go mugs with steaming fresh brew, then driven the eight hours and ten minutes to exit 401 off I-80 heading west to address 200 Campers Circle. The rear passenger door flung open before my father could even come to a stop. Dawn—a platinum blonde before I left, but now a chocolate brunette—sprang from the vehicle toward me. Upon colliding, she and I jumped in a circle, hugging and squealing in delight.

"You're here!" I jumped up.

"I'm here!" She jumped.

We had, in fact, been apart much longer than the four months that had passed since we last embraced. I stayed away for five months, six months, seven and a half months on my longest ship contract. But the time that had passed now felt different—more profound, expansive, and longer than the calendar cared to reveal. It could have said a year had passed, maybe two, and I'd have agreed.

I was elated to see her. She was, after all, my person. I tormented her well enough when we were kids, but now she was my first call. She cried when I moved to Colorado, then etched out a week in her life to come visit. She supported my decision to work at sea and then booked a trip on my ship. We danced in our pajamas all day Christmas Day and stayed in on Friday nights to watch movies. She was a great listener, but also, I never had to say much, which suited me. She alone was the one who found our mother at home, several hours into a grand mal seizure. She was there at Universal Studios when the ambulance came to take Mom to the hospital. She was fun to be around, and also, I never had to explain a damn thing. She had been there all along. She already knew.

"You're brown," I said, touching the ends of her shoulder-length hair.

"I am. Just a fun change. Do you like it?" She had been dyeing her hair since she was fourteen.

"You'd look good dressed in a paper bag," I said, quoting our father, and she laughed.

At the car, I wrapped my arms tight around my father's neck, then stooped at the front passenger seat to help my mother out. The floor was filled with its usual remnants—used Arby's napkins, crinkled grocery store coupons, a shiny gum wrapper atop a scrap piece of carpet as the floor mat. This was very much my father—taking care to protect the condition of something, like a car's interior with a durable covering, from who he knew himself to be—a man too overwhelmed to mind a mess.

"Hi," I said, grabbing under my mother's nearest arm and hoisting her to her wobbly feet. She steadied herself with her other hand upon the door frame.

"Hi." She grinned. She wore a polyester top embroidered with the charity's logo (a gift from Nate) and smelled of sweet cinnamon gum. I folded her into my arms and breathed her in. She smelled of home.

At the campsite, I took care to find the plushest, level patch of grass.

"I think here's the best spot," I said to Nate, telling him where we should place the tent. I bent down to my knees and began combing the blades, tossing sticks and shards of nature aside.

"Is that necessary?" he asked.

"How about you go inside and visit with my father?" I suggested without looking up from the grass. "Let me be with Dawn."

My father sat on the couch in the RV, enjoying the quiet while we busied ourselves with the tent. My mother was outside too, in a cloth folding chair with netted cup holders under the refreshing shade of a mature elm. The outstretched branches moved gently in the warm breeze.

Nate walked into the RV. Dawn joined me on the ground. "I really can't believe we're here. It's crazy to know you've run here—from San Francisco," she said, picking up a rock and tossing it aside.

"I know, right?" I tossed a twig.

"Like, Dad was driving for eight hours, and I kept thinking, *Ashley's going to run this!*"

"I know. Right?!" I looked at her with big eyes.

"Crazy," she said, shaking her head.

I moved on. "Here, hand me that bag."

She turned on her knees and grabbed the tent bag by the cord that cinched it closed at the top. Inside were its pieces—the canopy, a tarp, and rods that clanged together when I pulled everything out. We unfolded the tarp in tandem. It caught the breeze and crinkled as it opened.

"So what's it been like? How's Nebraska?" Dawn asked. "I feel like we hardly have time to talk."

"I know. I'm sorry," I said, laying the tarp on the ground. "It always feels like there's so much to do. And then when I'm not doing something, all I want to do is lie down and do nothing."

"Yeah, it's okay. I'm not trying to make you feel bad," she said. "Just... I'm here now, so tell me all the things."

I smiled. "Okay, well, Nebraska is great. The people here are so nice and welcoming. You'll see it this weekend. They're just so supportive."

I grabbed a rod from the pile. "Here, these extend like this," I said, pulling at each section and fitting them together. I handed her one. "The weather's been hot, you know, but it's not unbearable yet. It's just really warm on the road because of the heat from the asphalt, and there's never any shade. We've been waking up pretty early."

"Yeah, how's that going?" she asked.

"Eh. You know. Nate's still a night owl, but we're making it work. It's just what has to be done, ya know?"

"Any wedding plans yet?"

I worked a pole through the loops across the top of the tent. "Um, not yet. I honestly just haven't thought about it much. There's not much time, and it's not like we can pay for anything right now anyway."

"Mom and Dad'll help," she said. Mom was sitting right there, but we talked as if she wasn't. She had dozed off, her MS fatigue.

"I know. I know. We have some ideas. Just... we're waiting until after the run to really dive into the details."

"What about a date? Do you have one in mind?"

Each pole was fastened into place. She and I stood at opposite corners of the tent, working the same pole into the pins on each corner, to hold it in place. Half of the tent bowed up in an arch under the tension of the secure rod.

"I don't know. Next year sometime, I think." We worked our way to the opposite corners. "My whole focus has been the run and fundraising, so I don't know. It's like he proposed, and then we woke up the next day, and it was right back to this. We still have to get him a visa and a job and figure out where we're going to live. So, yeah," I said, securing the final pin into the rod, "there's a lot to figure out."

I sounded aloof, like I couldn't explain the budding of a plant to an inquisitive observer. Like I didn't know about the importance of nutrient-rich soil, adequate sunlight, and just the right amount of water. These things could've been at the top of my mind, but they weren't. My mind was a concrete path and painted lines. It was blogs I had little time to write, a Facebook post, a Twitter post, and a Flickr picture. It was what time I'd have to wake up to be done running and showered and to Omaha by the time the movie fundraising event started. It was a collection of unread messages in my inbox and an interview with the radio on the side of the road.

It was a twenty-dollar donation here and a five-dollar donation there, but not the $100,000 donation needed to get me to where I planned to be. It was when we'd move the RV next and where it was safe to park overnight. It was when to rotate my shoes, where to do the laundry this week, and how much recovery shake was left before we'd have to place another order. And then it was where to ship the order based on where I thought we'd be. My mind was all these things and more, making my plant a cactus, surviving off the showers of a springtime past. It was easy and durable. It'd have to wait out the drought.

"Looks cozy, babe," Nate called, stepping from the RV.

I turned to him and pointed. "That's because you don't know what you're looking at," I said with a smile. I stood up from the ground where I finished pounding in a stake and walked toward him.

"Come on," I said, touching his hand and giving him a kiss. "Help me grab some cushions."

We ate dinner that evening at Applebee's. It was close to the campground and was likely to have both bacon and fried onion rings for my mother. The five of us piled into my father's Malibu—my parents in the front, Dawn, me, and Nate in the back in that order—and drove the little ways to a packed restaurant parking lot. My father parked the car up front in a vacant handicapped spot, turned off the ignition, and hung their handicapped registration tag from the rearview mirror.

That their handicapped access was removable was deliberate. Like the car's floor mats, certain things came with intentional care. "We don't need her looking at a wheelchair on our license plate all the damn time," my father said about using the tag instead.

It was about the subtle message that that permanent image would send—that by looking at the wheelchair all the time, they'd accept that's what she would need.

Inside, we were seated at a large round table. My parents sat next to each other with their laminated menus propped up in front of their faces, sharing the no-prescription eyeglasses my father bought at Walmart for $1.34.

"Here, Beaner, get that other pair from your purse," my father said.

My mother bent down to the floor and hoisted the lug of a purse onto her lap. It was a chestnut faux leather handbag that weighed more than it needed to, considering that my father took care of everything. But still, it had some essentials—her photo ID (no longer a license but rather simply an ID card since it had been years since she was able to drive), a brick of a wallet filled with God-knows-what credit cards, and a couple of twenty-dollar bills, a plethora of fast-food napkins, cinnamon gum, her seizure medication, and, of course, an extra pair or two of cheap eyeglasses. She started digging.

"Here, gimme that thing," he said to her.

"I got it," she said, pulling the purse away, guarding what little independence she still had. A moment later, the eyeglasses emerged. "Here." She handed them over with a smile.

Instead of removing the first pair on his face, my father set the second pair atop. My sister and I looked at each other and then started laughing.

"What?" he said, peering over the edge of his makeshift bifocals.

"Nothing," she and I said in unison, still laughing.

His eyes went back to his menu. "You'll see," he said. "Someday. You'll see."

That evening, we ate together, much as we had in the past. My sister and I caught up, Nate and I told stories, my mother shared when she could, limited by her MS in both her ability to follow a conversation and also to speak in length, and my father didn't say much at all, mostly because he'd only been able to catch pieces of the conversations since he'd lost much of his hearing all those years ago.

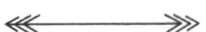

MY MOTHER ATE A BLT with a side of onion rings, both sizable (and messy) foods that she could mostly manage on her own. When it came time for her to sip her drink, my father would scoot the beverage cup with a bendy straw near the edge of the table. She'd drink, and then he'd slide it back out of reach, careful to clear it of her unsteady hands, lest they knock it over on their way to the sandwich.

When it came time for her to use the bathroom midmeal, even though we took her when we first arrived, I popped up to help.

"You got it?" Dawn asked.

I wiped my hands on my napkin. "Yeah, I'll go."

It was a willingness that hadn't always been there. To me, her incessant bathroom trips hadn't been connected to her MS until I learned that they were.

What did I really think? That she was doing this on purpose to bother me? Until I started the nonprofit, I didn't know that bladder dysfunction was a symptom of the disease. I'm not sure anyone told me. I'm not sure I was even listening.

I tucked my arm under hers and guided her through Applebee's toward the bathroom.

"Thank you," she said, staring in concentration at the ground.

"No problem, Mom," I replied gently at her side.

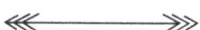

THE CITY OF YORK'S Fourth of July Parade was a celebration unlike any other in nearby towns. It marched along its main street, float after float, among a crowded street lined with hundreds of residents from near and far.

"You must be part of the parade," the City's Chamber Director wrote me via email. "It's the largest Fourth of July party from here to Iowa."

What that meant was lost on me. How big were other Fourth of July parties between here and Iowa? I didn't think to ask. It was a parade. It was the Fourth of July. We'd sit together—my dad, mom, Dawn, Nate, and I—in the car decorated with the charity's information and wave out the window. We'd spend the rest of the day eating and drinking. What else was there to know?

That I used alcohol in college to survive large gatherings of people would have been a helpful reminder, for one. That Nate would insist I walk outside the car to meet people would have been another.

"Nate, there's no reason we can't sit in the car and wave from the window."

"Babe, look at this crowd," he said, energized by the mass of people lining the street, five people deep, shouting and waving their tiny American flags. A fire truck roared its horn.

"You've got to walk alongside the car," Nate hollered. "Hand out your business cards."

He was jumping out of his skin.

A knot formed in my stomach.

"I don't even look like a runner," I said, looking down at my white T-shirt, cut-off denim shorts, and the cowboy boots I'd bought for myself back in Steamboat Springs. I wasn't thinking about representing the charity. I was thinking that it was the Fourth of July, that I'd sit in the car and then do what we always did, which was mosey around town eating a brat and drinking beer.

"I look like Daisy Duke."

"Babe, you gotta walk and wave. Just think about the donations." He was the liveliest I'd seen him in a long while.

I swallowed a lump in my throat and thought about that beer.

"We'll walk with you," Dawn chipped in. "Here, give me some cards."

Nate handed her a fat stack of cards and then took some for himself. He gave me the rest.

"Come on," he shouted, pulling at my wrist, smiling. "Like this." Then he dropped my hand and turned toward the crowd.

"She's running across America for her mum!" I heard him shout to a family over the noise, pointing back at me, handing them cards.

"She's running across America," he shouted to the next.

This is it, I thought. *This is why the fundraising trickled in dollar by dollar each month rather than in heaps. Because I wasn't more engaging, because I didn't rally a crowd.*

I could do some of it. I could talk to any runner or groups of them, especially if we were running. I could talk to the young girl who handed me her weekly allowance as a donation. I could stand in front of a crowd who knew what to expect, and I could speak, as I had earlier that week when a group of eighty people from the area running club showed up to hear my story and meet my mom.

But I couldn't do it all the time. I couldn't hand my card to the gas station clerk sitting there during their shift while we stopped in for ice cream sandwiches. I couldn't approach the woman returning her grocery cart at the same time as me. I couldn't bombard a crowd of families at a parade who were there to celebrate the floats.

"I don't get it," Nate would say later. "You should be telling everyone all the time. You speak so well to groups. I've seen you do it."

I looked at him, not knowing what to say. He was right. I didn't get it either. "I don't know, Nate. Sometimes I'm not ready. Sometimes, I just want to be a girl buying some ice cream."

"Well," he said, gesturing with his hands. Like, *Do you want to raise half a million dollars or not?*

Still, I didn't change. I didn't know I didn't have to. I wish I had known how powerful it is to be internal, that I could spend hours alone each day running down a highway and that it would deepen my ability to positively influence those around me and strengthen my presence, that it was okay to need time to transition from that space to social experiences, that it wasn't odd of me to be this way, that it was fine because it was me and this is how I was made.

I wish I could have said, "That's what you're good at. You do that, and I'll do this, and together, we make a great team." Instead, I felt small. I felt like I was failing. I felt like I wished he had never pointed it out to me in the first place.

Later that night at the campground, after the forced smiling and eating in York was done, after the fireworks exploded in a dark black sky and I felt loose on too much wine, I reached for my mother's hand. My father sat at the picnic table, talking with Nate. Dawn walked along the edge of the grass, chatting with her boyfriend on the phone. My mother and I sat near a crackling fire.

"Do you remember that time in high school?" I asked her.

"What time, honey?" She took a sip of her wine, a fermented rosé contained within a sealed travel mug set on her lap, a bendy straw poking out of its hole.

I stared at the glowing wood. "That time. When I was a freshman." My voice broke. "You know, when you were in the hospital for all those weeks?"

"Ashbee?" she said, concerned.

"I, uh, I just wanted to say I'm sorry," I said. I looked at her, and tears rolled down my cheeks. "That it took me so long to come by."

It was the thing I thought about most when I thought about regret. The way I ignored what was happening. The way I carried on like nothing had changed. A knowing woman asked me back in Utah, "What are *you* running from?" unable to accept that I would traverse a continent out of love, and I thought of this—my mother rebuilding her life in a hospital and me unable to stand at her side.

"Sweetie," she said, squeezing my hand, "you were just a kid. I had forgotten."

Looking into her soft eyes, I wondered if I ever could.

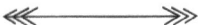

THANKFULLY, THERE WAS MORE running, and I needed it.

The next day, we awoke—my family from the motorhome, Nate and I from the tent that he got used to after I gathered up a nest of cushions—and we ran.

My route out of Lincoln took us east along a busy four-lane highway with a sidewalk. Dawn ran beside me, and my father biked while Nate drove the car with my mother. Then they'd switch. My father would drive, and Nate would run. Dawn would drive, and Nate would bike. I ran, always. And my mother, as she did, waved overenthusiastically from the car window.

We leapfrogged like this—from the campground to Superior Street, then northeast along Cornhusker Highway. Nate took pictures. My father took pictures. Dawn took pictures. The heat rose, and we decided to break, at which point Dawn, my father, and my mother all piled into the Malibu after we hugged goodbye and drove eight hours home to Wisconsin. I kept running.

Two days later, I crossed my fifth state line.

CHAPTER SEVENTEEN
Mad Summer

THEN, LIKE A MAD summer thunderstorm crashing a backyard BBQ, a storm rolled in, and everything changed.

"If you leave, there will be nothing for you to come back to!" I screamed at Nate under the shade of a giant oak at the edge of a beautiful Iowan farm ten days after crossing into Iowa.

The words erupted from the depths of me, boiling hot like the miserably humid days I now ran through. They weren't reckless; they were true. The words were a slow tide rising that buckled so suddenly that there was no fail-safe to stop them. Just... there it was. If Nate departed for Australia, as we argued over his doing so now, our relationship would be over.

My words hung in the air—thick and hot and angry. But true.

If I'm honest, I should have seen it coming. I would have, had I been paying any attention. Our relationship was not a cactus, after all. It was a leafy houseplant that needed regular care like any other leafy houseplant. Instead, I toiled upon the mountain of work I enjoyed being busy with, thinking that we enjoyed it together. Sure, we disagreed about money, but didn't everybody? That was normal, right?

My father had been collecting the mail being sent to the charity's PO box each week. Their home was the address listed on the nonprofit IRS application. Each day, they'd receive something for MS Run the US, and he'd collect it inside a shoebox I set by the front door, or so I hoped.

"Dad, you *have* to put all the charity's mail in this box," I said of the shoebox. "We can't lose any donations while I'm gone. Okay?" Their home wasn't a problem for the nonprofit until I left it. My father, with his hoarding and care of my mother, was always misplacing something.

On my way out of Lincoln twelve days ago, Dawn brought up the shoebox and its contents while running at my side. Nate glided along on the bike.

"Oh, I keep forgetting: Dad's got a bunch of mail for you," Dawn said.

"Great," I replied. "Any big checks?"

She replied with wide eyes, "Let's hope so."

Ten blocks later, Dawn, Nate, and I all came upon my parents, sitting in the parking lot of Casey's convenience store and gas station. At the open trunk, I tore into a juicy orange.

"Don't forget the mail," I said to Dawn.

"On it!" Dawn called from the back passenger seat.

Nate straddled the bike, chatting with my father.

I looked through the envelopes, opened neatly by my father with a letter opener. Some were check donations. Some were thank-you letters from people living with MS. Some were monthly giving statements from a faith-based radio station. I jammed everything but the checks and thank-you notes into the plastic grocery bag we used for a trash bin. A glob of banana peels browned inside the bag.

"What's that?" Nate asked, pointing to the papers.

"Some checks. A couple hundred dollars' worth," I replied, looking around for a dumpster.

"But what about these?" he said of the monthly giving statements I had crumpled up and tossed in the bag. He pulled one out.

"Oh, that's a monthly giving statement," I said.

"What do you mean 'giving statement'?"

"A giving statement," I said. "Like, a donation."

"A *donation*?" He repeated back. "You're giving money away?"

"It's not the charity's money," I said in defense. "It's from *my* bank account, obviously."

"Your bank account?" he repeated, again saying what I had just said back to me. "You're not *making* any money," he said, raising his voice. "Why are you *giving* money away if you're not *making* any money?"

That he was shocked and irritated fit within our recent conversations—about buying a tow dolly that I thought was unnecessary, about staying for free in random parking lots rather than paying for camping, about what we'd do for money when this was done. I held ground on decreased spending from the charity, yet here I was, continuing my monthly giving.

"It's for God," I explained. "I started it last year. I'm not going to stop just because I'm doing this."

"Don't you think doing this is enough?" he asked. "God doesn't ask for your twenty dollars a month if you're not making any income."

"It's an act of *faith*, Nate."

"It's irresponsible, Ashley. You have to cancel it. It doesn't make sense."

"No," I said firmly.

It didn't need to make sense. What about anything that had happened since Barcelona did? Those who loved me knew that my resolve was like the weather; there was nothing that could be done about it. I closed the trunk with a gentle *thud*.

"Now," I said, looking at him, "would you like to run with me again, or would you rather ride in the car?"

He glared at me for a moment and then turned toward the car. "I'll stay with your mum."

In the days that followed, my family departed, and I crossed over the Bob Kerrey Pedestrian Bridge from Omaha into Iowa, where the dense humidity of a sweltering Midwest summer settled in. It was a concrete transition—from workably warm days to thick, scorching air that punched me in the face like waves of heat from an oven. It made the relentless hills of Iowa and miles of vast corn fields grueling. Iowa had the topography of a jagged sawtooth, I found. Who knew?

I'd run up a hill, then back down a hill, then right back up another hill, and back down again. It went on for miles until a biker came alongside me and confirmed what my legs already felt.

"Oh yeah," he said, coasting for a bit, wondering why I was running along the highway. "Iowa is brutal. I've biked the whole thing, and you won't see a flat line until the Mississippi."

"All right," I said, considering the rise in front of me, now knowing it'd drop down the other side and continue doing so, rising and falling, up and down, for the next thirteen days. "Thanks."

Determined to beat the heat and those damn hills, I set my alarm so early the next day that I dragged Nate out of bed at 4:00 a.m.

He grumbled. I packed the car.

Out on the route, Nate remained trapped inside the car, too hot to open the windows and too drained to want to join me, and either way, the horse flies now swarmed and bit like the tiny bastards that they were if one stood still for too long. I'd find him napping in a reclined driver's seat or flipping through the worn pages of a book, the car idling, AC blasting, while I went on running, up the roads and back down, up again and back down, feverish out on the highway, all on my own in the dense hotness.

It was my greedy urgency for a distraction that led me to say yes, against my better judgment, to a runner from Des Moines when asked if we could run together after his work let out at 4:30 p.m. It'd be the hottest part of the day.

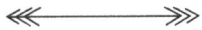

"AND HOW'S YOUR MOTHER doing?" asked Carl, the Des Moines runner I'd agreed to join. He bounded beside me on fresh legs in his sweat-wicking running attire while the sun blazed overhead in a cloudless sky, as it had been.

I ran along with him, pretending that my legs weren't trashed from the 168 miles of hill intervals I had just run in sweltering weather all week.

"She's okay," I said. "She has her good days and her bad days, but we're doing okay."

He was working his way through a series of common questions I had become accustomed to—*What do you eat? What kind of shoes are you in? What's your pace? When will you finish? How much money have you raised? How are you feeling? What's the hardest part? How's your mom?*—and I offered him the same response I gave to others, a watered-down truth.

They were lead—not the questions, but my legs, two hunks of unyielding metal bolted at my waist. We had only just begun our first of six miles together.

"Did you grow up here?" I asked, hoping to redirect the conversation.

"Yeah, actually," he replied. "North of the city. And then I moved closer to the capital when I got my job at…"

He went on, and I half listened, catching only snippets of conversation while I forced my arms back and forth, pulling my legs along. My heart hammered in my chest. My body trudged forward.

"And what's your favorite place been so far?" he asked, another question from the regular bunch.

"Right here, where I am," I replied, another answer from my regular bunch.

Until now, it had been true. I had been exactly where I had wanted to be, not wishing the journey away. Then I ran into Iowa, and my days became nothing short of a slog.

I iced myself—my knees, my feet, hell, even my *face* at the end of each run—and it offered marginal relief. The motorhome had become a dark cave, with its curtains drawn to keep out the sun while we blasted the AC overhead. Its jet-like hum drowned out the conversation I'd have had with Nate if I had had the energy to have a conversation.

Then, peeling myself off the bed, the couch, or the floor, I'd force myself out the door, like I had now, to run along the uneven sidewalks of Des Moines with Carl, feeling slowly boiled like a dumb lobster. It had been nearly two weeks of this. To give him the truth would have been to say I was ready to leave this unexpected hell behind.

"It's much hillier than I expected," I offered.

"I know! Most people assume it's flat, but it's actually quite brutal. I rode my bike across it for RAGBRAI. Are you familiar with it? It's a bike event across the state."

"I am, actually. A pack of RAGBRAI bikers stopped to chat a few days back. They told me all about it. Sounds cool."

"It is. You should do it sometime. They have aid stops in each city, and the people of each town really get into it. They have themed rest stops and bars offering drinks and..."

He continued on, and I tried to focus. *Drive your arms.* I told myself. *Breathe. Dig deep. You ran here from California. Now act like it.*

By now, into the second mile, I was less interested in deflecting conversation and more taken aback by how difficult it felt to run. My body felt heavy, as if I had filled my limbs and core with torrid sand.

Chills covered my skin.

Acid from my stomach crept up my throat like lava, threatening to show Carl my lunch.

"Let's stop for a minute," I said, interrupting whatever Carl was saying. I bent down with my hands on my knees.

"You okay?" Carl asked, concerned.

"Yeah. I just... I don't feel good," I said, wiping the sweat from my brow with a clammy hand. I stood, slightly hunching over, willing the food to stay put, and saw the motorhome parked on the side of the road near a gleaming golden dome.

"Let's get to the RV," I said.

At its threshold, I fell onto the steps and crawled inside its cooled core, lying myself face down across the floor.

"Babe, what's going on?" I heard Nate say above me.

"Ice. Water." My face was pulsing hot, ready to burst.

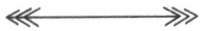

THE FOLLOWING DAY, IT wasn't the heat exhaustion that stuck with me. Rather, it was the event's ongoing lag in fundraising. Sure, I had almost puked. And honestly, my ego was a little bruised in front of Carl, who had to continue his run without me. I took a nap and rested. Then the next day, I awoke early to run, and everything felt fine. My mind rebounded back to its usual track—running, fundraising, awareness. I discussed my recent thoughts over lunch.

"You know, I bet we can find a runner to do this whole thing next year. Like, what if we're the charity that helps people run across America for MS fundraising?"

"How would that even work?" Nate asked.

I handed him his foot-long sub and placed mine at the seat opposite him. An unopened bag of potato chips crinkled in my hands. The AC unit roared overhead.

"I dunno. Runners keep saying that they've always wanted to do something like this. So, we could set it up so they can. The charity could supply the motorhome and care, and the runner would do the running and fundraising," I explained.

"How are we going to find one person to run across the country *and* raise enough to make it worth it?"

"I think there are runners who would want to do this," I said, unwrapping my roasted chicken sandwich.

"*We're* not even fundraising that much. How is someone else going to do it?" he replied.

"Okay," I agreed, "Maybe not one person. But a team could definitely do it. Like, each person has a week, and each runner has to fundraise to make the team. People could take a week off work to run across their section of the country. It would be like a destination event."

He bit into his meatball sub. "And who manages the event? We're not getting paid to do this. How are we going to pay someone else to do it?"

"Well, I was thinking we could crew together. You keep saying you don't know what you're going to do for work yet without a visa, and it'd be much easier with both of us. We could stay in the RV and take care of them together."

Nate set his sub down and took extra care searching for a chip from his bag. "We should just focus on this year and getting to New York for now."

I pressed on, as I do, outlining a vague dream that was rising within me, without knowing that I was actually naming what had become his nightmare—continuing to volunteer his time to runners on desolate highways across America, waking each day to sunrise mornings and permanent snack bitch. I was hyperfocused, having never been terribly attentive to others in the first place, on creating a completely new running experience and the excitement of raising more money. It wasn't difficult for me to miss his earnest dread at the thought.

"I mentioned it to my parents. They really liked the idea," I said, taking a bite of my juicy chicken-and-pepper-jack-cheese sandwich.

"You talked to your *parents* about it already?" he barked. "We have *none* of this figured out. We're not even to New York yet!"

"Okay. Geez. I just want to keep this going," I said. "I can feel it's what I'm supposed to do."

"What about me, Ashley?" he asked, looking at me. "What am *I* supposed to do?"

I thought I had answered that, thinking about his career and needing to wait for a visa anyway. But by the way he looked at me now, I realized it was more than that. To marry me, he'd leave his life in Australia—his family, his friends, and everything he ever built for himself to start anew with me. What were his options? How would I support him? That's what he was really asking.

I set my sandwich on its wrapper. "I don't know," I said, chewing. "What do you want to do?"

He looked out the window, past the wooden picnic table that came standard with our campsite, into the empty space beyond. "I'm not sure yet."

That he was unsure didn't feel like my problem. I couldn't figure out his life's purpose *for* him. Why couldn't we focus on mine until his sorted itself out? I listened and yet felt no onus toward what he was saying.

Instead, I thought of a girl like myself who could learn how to apply mascara with the help of her mother's steady, healthy hand. Of a girl who could go shopping with her mom because, though her father was endearing, hearing that "everything looks great" was actually no help at all. Of a little girl who wouldn't have to hear "Why does your mom walk like that?" one more time. I dreamed about actually doing something about this shitty disease, about helping in a way that made a difference.

What I hadn't considered was that this was my dream, not our dream.

Then, his visa extension was denied, and we screamed at each other under the shade of a giant oak at the edge of a beautiful Iowan farm.

"My visa is expired! I'm here illegally! I *need* to leave!" he yelled.

"*Need* to? You don't even *want* to be here!" I screamed back.

"Does what *I* want really even matter? Do I even get a choice?" he countered.

"Yes, like the fact that *you* chose to do this with me. I never forced you to!"

"Well, it's not *my* fault my visa is up," he said, blaming me, because it actually was kind of my fault—me, begging him to fly to the United States early on a six-month vacation visa because I missed him and thought there'd be no way the US would deny an Australian a visa extension. It was *Australia*, after all. A literal paradise.

"Babe, that means flying home in June. You'll still be running. That doesn't make sense," he stated.

"We'll figure it out," I encouraged. "It won't be a problem. It's not like you're from Mexico."

Yet it was a problem, kind of, depending on which one of us you asked. We were engaged to be married, so wouldn't that get him a permanent visa? Could he really imagine leaving his fiancée to run across America by herself?

The truth was that it wasn't actually the adventure we had imagined. He wanted me, but not like this. He wanted a break but wouldn't say it, and he couldn't take it, except now he had a perfectly good reason for it. He could return to Australia—he *had to*, of course, because he was here illegally. And he could work a job that would pay him, and see his family and his friends, and be absolved for just a moment of a mad woman running and all the nomadic camping. And then maybe I'd be me when he returned, except that I wasn't the me I used to be anymore.

Neither of us said what was really at the center—that this tour across the country was a lot of fucking work that had morphed from a short six-month adventure into a lifetime charity event.

So I screamed at him. And *that* is when the fantasy I conjured up of us doing this together evaporated, and I realized we were not a happy couple on a tour boat at the bottom of Niagara Falls, enjoying the flurry of rising mist together.

Rather, we were a set of ducks, teetering on a log, plummeting down the face of the falls into the roaring expanse below. As ducks, surely we would each survive. But the log that we traveled on would, without a doubt, be shattered into a million pieces, leaving us bewildered at the thought that we ever entertained it as a stable vessel to embark upon in the first place.

I needed his help, but he resisted giving it.

I wanted him here, but only on my terms.

Some things, like diamonds, are formed under pressure, while other things simply explode.

On the roadside.

Somewhere in Iowa.

And nobody knew a thing.

CHAPTER EIGHTEEN
Sloshing

SLOSH. SLOSH. SLOSH.

The ice in my hydration pack swished back and forth to the cadence of my steps—an audible *slosh-slosh-slosh-sloshing* my fury into muted unrest. I ran away from Nate and the giant oak tree. I had grabbed my pack and left.

I ran to cover miles. I ran to give us space. I ran, as I always had, to manage life and wondered all the while how I would do it if he left.

Could I drive both vehicles each day—park the car at the finish, drive the RV to the start, run between the two, and then use one vehicle to retrieve the other? I *did* have the tow dolly now. *And* my hydration pack so I could carry nutrition. And I *could* stash food and hydration along the way. I could do all that. The thought of it was ridiculous, but, fuck it, I would. I would run twenty-six miles each day, operate the organization, manage media interviews, and meet runners for the seventy-five days that remained. I, of course, first planned how to move on without him, because I wasn't needy or dependent. Not even this would stop me.

And then I thought about all the questions that would come. And they would. Our relationship was a public part of this story, and I cringed to think of the inquiries that I'd have to answer. They'd be constant. They'd make me actually *think* about how I felt.

Where's Nate?

SLOSHING

Why'd he leave?
Are you two still engaged?
How do you feel about it?

How do I feel about it? That was a great question. How *do* I feel about it? What would I say? The truth? That I, myself, too, couldn't believe he had left, thinking that it wouldn't be the end of our relationship, because what does it say about a partner to leave the other during the achievement of a lifetime? Was I absurd to think that the visa was a nonissue because we were engaged and our marriage would eventually make him a legal citizen?

It's not like Border Patrol was going to exactly try and find him within the next two months. It's not like he was a criminal. He was just drifting–not even taking a spot in the American economy. How would they even know how to find him before I finished? My parents hardly knew how to find us unless I gave them precise directions.

And, also, I wasn't *ready* for our relationship to be done. We had only just begun. The event was consuming, but it'd be done soon enough. *Is this how we are, or is it the event making us this way?* I wondered. The disagreements and the gray lines and the early mornings and the stifling, unbearable, torrid weather and the no personal space or time or money–it all kept piling up. And would it stop piling if we were under normal circumstances? I couldn't be certain. I was too close to the matter, like trying to view my fingerprint by placing my thumb to my nose. The details were too blurry; our form was beyond recognition.

Slosh. Slosh. Slosh.

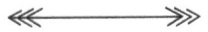

YEARS AGO, I ARRIVED home from a cruise ship tour to my parents' house filled with a mountain of stuff piled higher than I had ever seen. Random socks, dirty jeans, old newspapers, candy wrappers, family pictures, last year's partially dismantled Christmas tree, mom's medical needles, pill containers. Every surface was covered, filthy. There was so much layered up and across that only a single path cut through toward the kitchen and stairs.

"What the *fuck*?" I seethed under my breath. Then I started cleaning. We were hosting Thanksgiving dinner for extended family, and they'd arrive in two days.

Running now, down Highway 6 in Iowa, I recalled this memory and my father's hoarding–how it escalated along with my mother's disabilities. The piles he collected were the walls he'd built to protect himself from the life he'd once imagined, taken by her disease, and others who might criticize his care for her. His love was as vast as the open sky. But always considering her first fatigued him–the midnight wakings from soiled garments, hauling her body to the car just to get a carton of milk, poking her peachy flesh each day with injections in hopes to delay progression, wondering all along–if this is what delay looked like, what was next? He managed it all and seemed okay. He was happy, right?

But there *was* the hoarding. *And* the drinking. And that he had nothing for himself. I'm not sure he thought he needed it. Running and recalling these things, I couldn't deny that ignoring one's needs for another only manifests a mess.

There was the running, and the questions, and the memories, and the sloshing.

An open road. *Slosh, slosh.*

A white line. *Slosh, slosh.*

A hot sun that blazed. *Slosh, slosh.*

The rhythm of running lulled my temper, like rocking a baby, and I softened.

Nate was here. And maybe he didn't do exactly as I expected, but maybe I was expecting too much, ignoring him too much? Maybe he did need a break, and who was I to tell him he didn't? But did he have to leave the country to get it?

After the running and the sloshing subsided. After he came for me in the car. After our eyes met, I confessed.

"You can't leave," I begged him selfishly. "I love you. Our marriage will make you legal."

We hugged, and he agreed. "Okay," he said. "But I can't do this by myself any longer. We've got to ask others to help."

SLOSHING

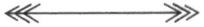

HELP.

A simple request.

If only it were that easy.

If only I thought needing help wasn't weak. If only I had seen my parents model it, because to do anything with my mother without my father there was nearly impossible—we practically had to pry her from his vice grip.

Nobody could care for her like he could, and she was his responsibility, he said. What if something happened to her while he wasn't there? He couldn't live with it. He wouldn't. In recent years, to take her to lunch, to get a pedicure, to sit at Starbucks for a few hours, to get her out and give him some space, my father would fetch my mother's purse and open it up.

Inside, he'd pull out a clear plastic case the size of a large wallet. Then he'd hold it up and say, "This is her seizure medication. If you think she's having a seizure, don't call the ambulance. It's not worth it. They'll do the same exact thing and charge us thousands. What I need you to do is pull down her pants, put the tip of the dispenser into her anus, administer the meds, and then hold her butt cheeks together so the fluid doesn't come out."

I'd nod and grab the plastic case. "I know, Dad. Don't worry. We'll be back in a few hours, okay?"

And then, finally, after he conceded and hired home aid help, of course, there was an issue.

"Do you see this?" my father said, holding up a receipt from KFC. "That woman got herself a roasted chicken and mashed potato meal, and only got your mother some cheapy chicken nugget box." He shook his head, crumpling up the receipt. "Not gonna happen."

That was the last we saw of home aid, and proof to my father that he could do it best.

So, was I asking too much of Nate? That he be out here with me exploring the American countryside while we traveled from one state to the next while not having to pay for it? Was it so hard that I should have to ask others to help too? I stared at my blank computer screen while these things swirled around in my mind, thinking of what to write on the charity's blog.

"So, what are you going to say?" Nate asked, staring over my shoulder. It was the day after the fight, and I promised I'd write a post right away to ask for help so Nate could take a break.

And yet. The fight was still raw. I couldn't unfeel how I felt. I ran and felt more empathy, and then I slept, and the fire roared again. How could he think that leaving might be okay?

"I'm not sure yet," I said honestly. "I think I'll run first."

So I did.

I laced up my shoes and went—hard at first to burn through the fire, and mile after mile, its raging dimmed. The calm came, and I enjoyed myself because I was running, and I could, and I did. I ran until my legs were tired and my stomach was empty and my lungs needed to rest. I ran until my ego was quiet and my pride felt foolish and love was a thing of compromise. I was no longer skipping from one guy to the next. I was committed. No one was perfect, and Nate was funny, kind, and good, and those things were plenty. I could ask for help for him. He had done so much for me.

What came out when I wrote was a vague picture that compared our recent fight to a hurricane. I alluded to differences but skipped over the details. Every relationship had differences, right? I could offer that. I gave readers an opaque view of what had actually occurred, hoping to distract those watching with analogies and a feeling of resolution. We were at a resolution, right? Someone just had to come out and help.

I hit Publish and then closed my computer and waited.

Everything since crossing into Iowa felt hard.

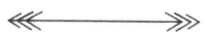

A WEEK AND A half later, I departed Iowa across the Arsenal Bridge. It spat me out into Illinois and down a road that quickly made me feel on edge. A dark, plastic bag of empty Bud Light cans spilled out onto the sidewalk. A condom wrapper lay discarded. I ran around it, giving it a wide berth, when out of my peripheral, a vicious dog came sprinting from the side of a small house.

I stopped and stood, stunned. The dog was fast and aggressive, and I was unable to comprehend what to do. It was the first time in all my running that a dog had come at me on the attack. My heart jumped into my throat as the creature lunged at me.

Just then, a chain-link leash yanked taut around its neck, jarring it to a stop at the edge of its lawn. It barked and growled, whipping foamed saliva from its teeth.

I released the breath I didn't realize I was holding.

Nerves pricked up my spine to the back of my head.

I took a step back, then another, looking over the house at the two front windows covered in sheer drapes, wondering if the owner was watching this interaction from behind them. I turned quickly and ran away.

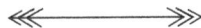

I CAME UPON THE dog after crossing the great Mississippi River via the bridge that connected downtown Davenport to Moline. Like running the Rocky Mountains may have felt if I had grown up there, crossing the massive, monumental river felt significant to me. I looked down at its brown, swirling current from above and felt nostalgic.

Not only was it a prominent geological milestone that benchmarked my continued progress and the end of the grueling Iowan hills, but it also weaved its way in and out of my entire life.

It was the river my mother learned to waterski on—her family having spent summers on their houseboat, pulling her up and down the waterway on a pair of polished planks. I recalled the Polaroid photos I found of her doing this in an album when I was fifteen—the way I stared at them, wondering what she was like, this slim, athletic version of my mother I would never know. It played a hand in how my father fell for her—him watching her "pop out of the water like a cork" all those years that they spent on her speedboat, beers and cigarettes and sunshine in hand.

It lined the town of La Crosse, Wisconsin, where I went to college. I ran over it many times then, too many to count, when I'd leave the worn and cracked blue house and make my way to the Cass Street bridge, over the moving river, into Minnesota, and back. My junior year there, it'd take the life of Steph's dear friend—when we'd paper the town for two days with fliers looking for him, until finally he was found washed up on its bank. Each time at the river thereafter, I morbidly wondered what that must have been like—for him to drop below the surface, desperate to rise but sinking instead, frantic for air, until at last he breathed in liquid and drowned. And for that person to find him—days later, grayed and bloated, lifeless upon its shore.

I thought of the drowning now, and all of it, as I ran across the massive waterway into Illinois. There was much to think about. My father had called a week and a half prior, almost immediately after I published the blog.

"What's up, kiddo? What can we do?" he asked through the phone.

"I dunno, Dad. Everything's really tough right now." I took the call alone, slipping outside the motorhome to walk around the campground in Des Moines. Arid dust kicked up from the parched gravel beneath my feet. "Nate needs a break. Do you think you and Mom could come out for a bit?"

"I'll talk to your mother. I'm sure we can make it work," he said. "Your brother can manage the grass. He owes me some hours. How much time you thinking?"

I felt grateful and small, like a child, like Nate and I couldn't manage this grown-up thing on our own. "I dunno. It's really up to you. Maybe. Could you do like a week or so? Just enough to give Nate some downtime?"

My father decided it would be three—my parents would crew me through what would remain of Illinois (after I arrived in Chicago), Indiana, and part of Ohio, and Nate would stay at their home.

"It'll be great!" my father encouraged me over the phone. "Your mother and I are really looking forward to it. You're doing real good, kid. Keep it up."

I breathed a sigh of relief. My parents wanted to come. *They were looking forward to it.* My father would drive—he loved driving, And my mother would wave overenthusiastically from the window, as she does, and of course, she would love that too. It'd be an adventure for both of them, for all of us. It would be great, just as my father had said. They *wanted* to come, and that wanting came to me like the refreshing sign of spring after a brisk, dreadful winter. I couldn't be so hard to take care of, could I?

I'd have my answer to that question in about 470 miles, which is what remained between that phone call and Chicago—eighteen marathons and tip-toeing through days with Nate. I ran gingerly, eager to pacify any irritants between him and me with an upbeat attitude, eager to prove how easy I was to care for, eager to show how simple this all really was. Which, actually, was not that simple when I considered what was ahead of me and the planning that had to be done for the myriad events surrounding my brief homecoming to Milwaukee while I ran through the region.

Just as quickly as I cleared the Rockies, people had begun to ask, "Are you coming home?"

My direct east route didn't take us through Milwaukee, but I had learned from the days and miles (and tension) I added to the event when I insisted I run to Salt Lake City that no one cared how I arrived off course. And so, I told them yes—I'd visit Milwaukee for a few days, 124 miles north of the running route, and to get there, we'd drive.

A few days in Milwaukee turned into four and then quickly tumbled end-over-end into a collection of appearances and fundraising events—a two-day, 150-mile bike ride with the MS Society, another fundraising event with Marcus Theaters, and a massive tailgating get-together at Miller Park on August 10, where I had been invited by the Milwaukee Brewers to throw out the first pitch.

I managed the needs of these events in between a fifteen-mile morning run and an eleven-mile evening run, after a stop at the grocery store, or on the highway during a walking break. I ran, I ate, I napped, and I replied—keeping myself very busy, busy, busy. It all was welcomed—a messy, purposeful distraction from other thoughts that threatened to take space in my mind.

"And how much square footage of the parking lot are you going to need?" the Miller Park event manager asked me over the phone.

I took the call, now showered and full, perched at the dinette in front of my computer after a humid and sunny seventeen miles near Newton, Iowa.

"Umm, I'm not sure," I said, blowing out air. "How much square footage do people usually get?"

"Well," she said, "it depends on how many people are coming. What's your attendance?"

"Umm, I'm not sure," I said again, feeling unprepared. "Can you tell me what kind of things you need to know, and then I'll figure out those things and call you back?"

"Okay, well, your attendance will affect the square footage we give you, which will affect how many tents, tables, and chairs you rent from Karl's Party Supply."

"Oh, we don't need a tent," I said. (Though, really, we did. The event was to start at noon in mid-August. We could count on it being *at least* eighty-five degrees if it were sunny, which it would be, and heat intolerance was a common symptom of MS, which many people in attendance would have. I had considered none of that.)

"Yes, you do," the woman said. "It's part of the event contract. We have a partnership with Karl's Party Supply. You're required to get the tent from there if you want to host an event in our parking lot."

"Okay, um. Do they donate tents for fundraising events? Or how does that work?" I asked. I bobbed my foot up and down anxiously. Nate, sitting across from me, looked at my foot, then looked at me. I stopped.

"Not exactly," she said. "It's $671 per tent, and that includes set up and take down."

"It's $671?" I asked. That was a week's worth of fundraising. That was 144 miles worth of running. I didn't even know how many people were going to come.

"Yes, that's correct."

"Okay, are you sure we can't just forgo the tent this one time? The Brewers invited me to throw out the first pitch because I'm running across America for my mother, and we're a very small nonprofit. We're completely volunteering our time to do this so that one hundred percent of what we raise can go toward research for a cure."

"I'm sorry," she replied, not seeming very sorry at all. "It's a part of the event contract."

"All right, well, is there any way you can give me a nonprofit rate or something?" Sounding desperate.

"Ma'am," she replied, exasperated with me. "This *is* the nonprofit rate."

I got off the phone and exhaled a puff of air from my lips.

Nate looked up. "You okay?"

"Yeah," I said, not feeling okay. "We're going to have to get a party tent."

He nodded, letting out a soft sigh. "Yeah, I heard." He knew how stressed I was about saving every dollar we could for the research donation. "I'm sorry."

I groaned. "I hate this. I just wish I knew who was coming and how much we're going to raise so I could justify the costs. It could be a total flop. What if no one comes?"

"Babe, people will come," Nate encouraged. "You just have to keep inviting them. Tell as many people as you can! They'll come."

"I know," I said, feeling down. "I am." I sat back with my hands behind my head and blew out another deep breath of air. Event management was not my strength. Creating a party experience to die for wasn't either. Running was. Being alone for five hours each day while trekking my ass down the highway seemed to be a pretty good fit too.

"Montel's flying in from New York," I said, putting my forehead in my hands. "What if people don't show? How fucking embarrassing."

"Let's shake this off," he suggested, "C'mon. Let's throw the ball around."

Outside, on an open stretch of lawn near our campsite, we tossed a baseball back and forth to each other.

"How far is it from the plate to the mound?" Nate asked, holding the ball in his hand.

"I don't know," I replied. "Hold on. Let me look it up."

I pulled my BlackBerry from its purple holster clipped to my shorts and typed in "Distance from MLB home plate to pitcher's mound" into the web browser.

"Sixty feet, six inches," I said.

"All right, let's measure it out," Nate said, walking toward me. He stood at my side and lobbed me the ball, then walked away from me, counting to sixty out loud. He wanted to make sure my pitch made it to the plate. He had grabbed a baseball at Walmart the week before so we could practice.

"All right," he said when he got to sixty and turned around. "You think you can make it this far in front of thirty-five thousand baseball fans?"

"Honey, I'm a tomboy. I can pass a spiral football. I have no problem throwing you this baseball," I replied, reiterating what I had said to him at the store while we stood in front of a bin of balls.

"But in front of a full stadium of people?"

I took the ball in my hand and sailed it through the air, getting it to him with both accuracy and distance. Even in a stadium full of people, I was sure of this. He threw it back to me. I caught it and sailed it back to him again. Back and forth we went, each throw coming with the sense of ease that can be expected after one spends years building muscle, proper motion, and movement memory. I threw the ball back again. He caught it right at the mark.

If only everything were this simple, I wished.

Later that afternoon, we gathered what we needed for the miles that remained for the day. I stuffed a fruit and nut granola bar into one of the hydration pack pockets and filled the bladder with ice cubes and cool water while Nate gathered up snacks, the camera, and his latest book, The Next Trillion, a read about upcoming mega wealth in the wellness industry.

"So I was thinking about the attendance number for the tailgate." His back was to me, placing five oranges in a food sack on the table.

"Yeah?" I replied. I folded over the silicone hydration bladder and slid on the plastic piece that secured the water inside.

"Let's just start a list," he said. "I'll bring the notebook, and whenever we think of someone, we'll write it down."

"Yeah. Okay," I said, taking a seat on the couch. I grabbed a clean pair of socks folded into each other and worked one on over my foot. "I'll send an email out tomorrow to everyone on the list, asking for an rsvp. We can start there, I guess."

Nate moved toward the door. The camera bag hung over his shoulder on the same side that held the grocery bag of snacks. The hand that held the book reached for the car keys.

"You still seem pretty down about it," he said. "I just don't understand. You speak so well in front of a crowd of people, like you did in Omaha, but then when you're one-on-one or need to personally invite people, you get all clammy."

He stood by the doorway, ready to go. "It doesn't really make sense to me."

I pulled on the other sock and then slipped my foot into my Asics, saying nothing, not knowing how to explain something I didn't understand myself. I stood up from the couch and gave him a shrugging look, then followed him out the door. The metal steps clanged and creaked as we descended.

"It's not that hard, babe," he continued, closing the door behind me and locking it. "All you have to do is ask."

In the Camry, driving on Highway 6 just east of Grinnell, toward where I'd start running, I peered out the passenger window at vast, lush prairie fields. The newest upbeat hit of the summer, California Girls, bobbed through the radio. So much depended on people showing up—from the $1,600 worth of T-shirts I bought for merchandise to Montel Williams flying in for the event, to the party tent we'd now have to pay for.

Klement's Sausage was donating three hundred hot dogs for us to sell. Would three hundred people show up? Who would sell them the hot dogs? What would Klement's think if there were hundreds of leftovers? My skin prickled over the worry that it'd be a small turnout. I couldn't help but feel as if I were passing my secret crush a note in front of the entire school: Do you like me? Check yes or no. My throat tightened.

At the spot on Highway 6, my feet hit the concrete, and I ran. One mile in, and already the grip let up. My shoulders dropped, my throat opened, and without me even noticing, the prickling disappeared. I breathed. I sweat. Mile after mile, I resurfaced. While everything else pulled at me, I had this—the release of running. So when I ran across the Mississippi River, nine marathons after the fight in Iowa, and halfway to our Chicago destination, I felt like I had achieved something, though I couldn't exactly name what.

My relationship with Nate, and the run as I knew it, threatened to cave in on itself. It meant something for us that it hadn't, right? That I had made it to this great Midwest milestone was another indicator that, despite it all, I made progress. I ran, feeling a significance I couldn't identify and the weight of all the things the river meant to me. Then I came upon the beer cans and the dog, and less than a mile later, Nate at the car.

"Babe," he said, standing on the curb near the trunk. "We're in Illinois."

He was elated. Was it because he felt the achievement of it too? Or was it just one day closer to his break?

"We're here," I said, giving him a high five. I was elated too. "Hey, let's find a place to camp for the night. I think I'm done for now."

"Everything okay?" he asked. It was still early. I could easily run more.

"Yeah. There was this sketchy street where a dog ran at me," I explained. "I just need a minute."

He stepped closer, knowing it wasn't like me to stop. "Are you okay? What happened?"

"Yeah, yeah. I'm okay," I said, not wanting to make it a thing. "It was on a leash, thank God. But for a moment, I didn't see that it was. These bigger cities may be less safe than out west."

He nodded like he was glad to finally see a rational side of me. "Okay," he said, scanning the street behind me as if he'd see the dog and do something about it. "Yeah, okay. Let's go. You know, I was thinking we should scout out the streets a bit more anyway, around Chicago and these bigger cities. I'll talk to your dad about doing it when we get to Milwaukee."

SLOSHING

He'd talk to my dad about doing it. I took off my pack and got in the car.

We opted for a campground twenty miles east of Moline, then another one two nights later near a place called Walnut, then Triumph. Each stop was a leap toward Chicago, which, for me, had become a destination in and of itself—a place to get to.

Somewhere, I imagined, the shadow of Nate wanting to leave and my failure to understand why would up and go away. He would rest, and all would be restored—back to the way it was, back before I was paying attention.

CHAPTER NINETEEN

Worth It

THE NAME *ASHLEY* IS an Old English surname that translates to "dwelling near the ash tree"—a fact that, as a preteen, felt uninspiring to me. *Dwelling near the ash tree?* I was hoping for something a bit more powerful.

Was I someone who'd felt like a dweller to my parents when they'd decided to name me? I had been a tiny little human in my mother's belly, already becoming who I was meant to be, and surely they must have been thinking of some significance when choosing my name. I mean, it's the *naming* of something.

"Oh, you know. We just liked the sound of it, kiddo," my father had told me when I'd asked him about it. I'd left the inquiry knowing it didn't really mean anything, and yet, I'd wondered about it—what it meant for me and my future—to be someone who would be found under the shade of a tree, dwelling there on a lazy and bright summer afternoon.

That I was born and raised in Wisconsin comes from my surname, Kumlien, of Swedish origin. My ancestor, Thure Kumlien, had crossed the Atlantic by boat as a naturalist explorer who had been meant to marry a socialite but had run away with the help instead—so the story goes. He'd discovered a never-before-discovered flower and an arctic bird. He'd settled in Milwaukee, Wisconsin, and become a professor. One hundred years later, here I am.

Milwaukee. Why? I'd wonder when I thought of Thure, my adventurous ancestor, to whom I felt a kindred connection. I'd done similar as he—discovered things, crossed great distances, done as I'd seen fit rather than what was expected of me. But maybe if he had known what was farther west, the great Rocky Mountains, then maybe I'd have been a Colorado native. Or maybe even just a bit farther to the south, and my mom wouldn't have had MS—being that the farther one lived from the equator, the higher the risk of diagnosis. But here we were. The Kumliens had settled in Milwaukee.

In high school, I'd steady myself on excursions to Milwaukee from the suburbs—readying myself to drive through what felt like a maze of complex, one-way streets, and happily bypassing it, with all of its on- and off-ramps, to and from the airport.

The city hadn't changed much at all since I'd left it for San Francisco, but as I arrived from Chicago in the motorhome, it certainly felt smaller. Looking at Milwaukee through the windshield, I knew which one of us had changed.

Heading north on I-94, Nate and I towed the Camry behind the camper in the center lane. We had long since learned our lesson of stop-and-go merging if we stayed in the right lane and knew better than to sit our vehicle at a top speed of sixty-five miles per hour in the fast lane. Driving the rig wasn't even a thought—like a limb that had grown from us that we easily maneuvered through Friday afternoon traffic. To our right, we passed an ornate church at National Avenue and, shortly thereafter, the Mural of Peace. Then, the view opened up to a panorama of the city's iconic Hoan Bridge and its massive Lake Michigan waterfront. Sunlight sparkled off the water. Sailboats tipped gently in the breeze.

"Babe," Nate said, looking at it with his mouth open. "That could be the ocean!"

I smiled, delighted that he approved. He had arrived in Milwaukee in November and had left with me in early March, having never enjoyed the pleasure of a perfect Wisconsin summer day—grilling brats, drinking beer from the cooler, and loading up the boat with refreshments and floaties. But now here we were on a bright and warm August day, perched up in the motorhome's driving quarters with a perfect view of the water that stretched beyond our sight to the north, east, and south. Near it, a cluster of high-rise buildings hugged the shoreline, making up the profile of Milwaukee's downtown business district. I had to admit, it felt welcoming.

Veering west, we passed Menomonee Valley, where a strong, organic smell of brewer's yeast—a local staple—filled the cabin, and shortly thereafter, Miller Park to the left. Four days from now, I'd be there at our tailgating event, throwing out the first pitch. We drove past the Petit National Ice Center, where I'd run my first marathon race—ninety-four laps indoors around the ice rinks in January—a weekend of races just a month before departing for the start, and farther still, past pitches of fields where I'd spent a decade playing youth soccer. Taking these places in, I was amazed at what I hadn't known the last time I'd been here. It felt like it had been years. It had only been four months.

On we went until we arrived at Brookfield—not at my parents' exit but at the one before it at our hotel, the Brookfield Inn and Suites, where we had a room.

Nate pulled the caravan of vehicles to a stop across two parking spaces and killed the engine. We walked inside empty-handed to check in, leaving our bags in the RV.

"Hi there! Welcome to Brookfield Inn and Suites! Checking in this afternoon?" a woman behind the counter greeted us.

"Yeah. Uh, my friend Matt is the Director of Sales, and he booked us a room under my name, Ashley Kumlien," I told her. "K-U-M-L-I-E-N."

"Sure. Great!" she said, clicking across the keyboard. "Yup. Ummmm. Yup, here we go." *Click, click, click.* "A room with two queens on the seventh floor. Sound about right?" She looked up from the computer screen with a big smile.

"Yeah, that's great," I replied, "I left the reservation up to him, so yeah, that's great."

Nate nudged my side. I looked at him, and he nodded toward the receptionist. He mouthed, *Tell her.*

"Yeah, uh, actually, it's a gift," I said, clearing my throat. "I'm running across America for multiple sclerosis, and Matt wanted to help out our charity, so he offered us a room here."

"Wow. Wait. What? You're running across America?"

I told her all the things—that my mom had been diagnosed with the disease, that I had started in San Francisco on March 22, that I had been running essentially a marathon each day for four months straight, that I had gotten as far as Chicago, and that I was from Brookfield so we were in town for a few days for fundraising.

"Honey, wow. That is just amazing. I can't hardly believe it," she said, shaking her head. She was middle-aged and had manicured nails and a billowing blowout atop her head. There was a good chance she either had a kid my age or knew someone who had MS who she didn't know about. Probably both. "So tell me about these fundraising events you're doing in town."

Walking back out to the motorhome to get our bags, Nate practically jumped on my back. "See!" he said, leaping around. "See? You just gotta do it! You did great! That was great! Do you feel great?" He was so proud.

I felt good. She had been receptive, taken my business card, and said she'd share the fundraising events with her friends. But I wouldn't describe how I felt as "great." There was a lump lodged in my throat, and to be honest, I wouldn't have said a thing if Nate hadn't nudged me to after the many conversations we'd had about me needing to do so.

I had told her about the event just now, but for the next four days, I'd be walking through the hotel lobby. What if she worked here every day? Would it be expected that I stop and talk to her each time? How do people who host fundraising events act once they've extended an invite? What if I wanted a beer at the restaurant bar? Would she find it odd that a girl running across America for charity was drinking a beer?

Sometimes, I felt bright and courageous, and these interactions just burst out of me with a confidence I could hardly control. These were the opportunities I'd use to email Montel or make a call to borrow a motorhome or walk into a running store to see if they'd donate shoes. But sometimes, I turned inward, as if each conversation were a mountain—and I could only climb so many mountains in one week. Still, Nate's excitement was endearing. I nudged him away from me jokingly as he leaped, and I smiled.

"Yeah, I know. I know," I admitted. "You were right. That was great."

In our room on the seventh floor, I set my duffel bag and backpack down on one of the two queen beds and pulled the curtains open to a vacant parking lot below. Though I could see the interstate and the mega mall to the north, the sound of whirling traffic was muffled by an insulated window and the tops of fluffy maple trees. What filled the room instead was the air conditioning unit humming to life at my knees and the sound of Nate turning on the TV. He flopped himself down on the open bed and propped one hand behind his head.

I sat on the other bed next to my bags. "So, I think we have about an hour or so before we should get moving to Wheel & Sprocket. The shop closes at seven, but the bike fitting will take about thirty minutes or so."

"Yeah, I was thinking," he said, staring at the TV. "I think I might just stay here. I kinda just feel like bumming around. Sleeping in. Watching sports. Maybe working out in the fitness center."

"Oh, okay," I replied. I hadn't expected him to skip the bike ride. The MS Bike 150, the two-day biking event that I had been invited to as an honorary guest, was the following morning at nine. When I'd been asked to attend a month ago, Nate and I had rallied over the idea of biking together. Finally, neither one of us would crew. Instead, we'd enjoy the event side by side, bonding over sweat and an endurance experience together. Then again, that had been before we'd fought beneath the shade of a giant oak tree.

"I thought you wanted to get out and exercise with me? You know, not sitting around in the car anymore waiting for me. Right?"

"Yeah, I dunno," he said with a little chuckle, finally looking from the TV toward me. "I can exercise here. I'd just rather not set an alarm tomorrow."

"Okay, yeah. No problem!" I said quite cheerfully, pacifying my surprise and disappointment with a bright attitude. "I'll just ask my dad!"

WORTH IT

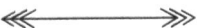

TWO HOURS LATER, DAD and I stood side by side at the Wheel & Sprocket bike shop in West Allis.

"Woah. Meister," he said in awe, using one of his many nicknames for me. Before us, the shop worker had propped up two sleek road bikes, both a glossy cherry red. The employee had then walked off, saying over his shoulder that he'd be right back.

The shop was busy, full of riders milling about with a buzz of energy. I knew it well. It was the stirring of adrenaline that came as an athlete prepared for an event. Wheel & Sprocket sponsored the two-thousand-person MS ride, and everyone was hustling to finalize last-minute details. We were here because they'd graciously offered to loan Nate and me a set of bikes so we could ride.

"Are these good?" I asked, clueless about the bikes before us. My father was a casual cyclist. He'd cycled first as a preteen paperboy and then, more regularly later, before marriage, on the miles of paved paths that spiderwebbed throughout the city of Milwaukee.

"These are amazing!" he said, easily picking up one of the bikes with a couple of fingers by the frame.

"They're some of the best we have," the worker said, returning to us. "These are the Trek Madone. They're light, strong, and extremely efficient. You two should have a great ride."

I could tell by his presence that he loved all things cycling, like the way he immersed himself in it now. Rows of bikes and frames without wheels hung from the walls throughout the entire shop. Tire racks were situated here, and replacement tubes and parts were gathered over there. Specialty helmets, clip-in shoes, fingerless gloves, water bottles—all of it—could be found somewhere within the shop, and he knew exactly what he was looking for and how to find it. Fitting us with these things was something he enjoyed.

"What's one of these run?" my dad asked while the man adjusted the saddle on my father's bike. "You know, if I decide to keep it."

The guy tilted his head back and forth, "About twenty-five hundred, give or take, depending on the accessories."

My father let out a low whistle and looked at me.

"These are nice, kid," he said with a smile. Then he floated out of the bike shop, wheeling a cherry-red frame at his side. And for the first time in a long time, I felt light too. At least I could give my father this. His excitement accompanied us to the event the next morning.

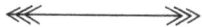

"AND WITH YOUR HELP," the event emcee bellowed into the microphone, "we *will* have a world free of MS!"

The crowd cheered, cyclists and spectators alike, clapping and hollering. My father and I clapped and hollered too. We stood straddling our bikes, one foot on a pedal, one foot on the ground like human kickstands in a sea of others doing the same. An hour prior, we had checked in at biker registration.

"Nate and Ashley?" the woman had asked, looking at me and my father.

"Nate couldn't make it." I lied. "I'd like to change his registration. This is my father," I said, hooking my arm into his and hugging it. He wanted to be here. I realized now, more than anything, that I wanted him here too.

The emcee finished the speech and began a countdown. My father and I pushed off with the crowd.

We moved slowly at first, hopping along. We teetered upon our frames at a slothful pace while a mass of speedy cyclists dispersed down the barricaded city street. Then we were off too, behind the lead cyclists, with many behind us, on a seventy-two-mile course that started us in Pewaukee and would snake us through miles of Southeastern Wisconsin farmland before finishing for the day in a city southwest of us called Whitewater. Within the first mile, we biked next to the lake where I'd run my first marathon from my parents' house the year before.

"You're the one running across America, right?" a gentleman said to my right.

"I am!" I said, smiling.

"So, what are you doing here?" he joked.

"Ha! I'm running through Chicago right now," I explained, "We have some fundraising events in the area, so the chapter invited me to ride while I was in town."

"Hey, she's with us!" a man flanking my father on the left said.

"Ah, Chuck. You always get the young, ambitious ones!" the man to my right joked. "My team's coming for you!"

"You're welcome to try," Chuck bantered. "But you're going to have to show up with more than just that *change* you brought last year."

At that, they both laughed.

For years, Chuck had remained the top fundraiser of the ride and was well-known throughout the organization for his fundraising fortitude. He'd gotten his start thirteen years before I would even think to run across the country. At the time of his diagnosis, he'd been an athletic thirty-five-year-old father of two. He'd gotten double vision one day while pitching softball and had found that it meant he had MS. The diagnosis had shaken him to the core.

Riding in this event—raising hundreds of thousands of dollars and razzing others to try and beat him in a friendly competition for the cause—was his answer to the merciless nature of the disease. Would he always be able to ride? Or would he be sidelined by debilitating symptoms? Doing everything he absolutely could right now was his productive way of sweating through the pain and making an impact. I could relate.

"Okay, so what's the secret?" I asked him now, riding at his side along a wooded suburban road that lined the lake's north shore. The morning was already warm. A breeze cooled my face. "How do I raise half a million dollars?"

"Well, that depends," he said, smiling. "Are you riding for my team or not?"

"Next year. For sure," I said, smiling back. "Promise."

He raised his hand, and we high-fived.

"Okay. Joking aside, it's a lot more than just sending a blanket email or posting on Facebook. You have to go old school. You have to shake some hands. You have to put a face to the disease and show your donors how you're swinging hard to make a difference."

"I feel like I'm doing that," I replied honestly, playing with the shifters and pedaling to get acquainted with the gears. "I just haven't seen the big donations come in yet."

Coming into Milwaukee, I had managed to raise nearly $40,000 in total. This sum was so far from my fundraising goal that I knew that raising half a million dollars would mean that someone very wealthy would need to get behind my story, or the run would need to go viral. Likely, I'd need both.

"What's gotten you into the big numbers?" I asked.

"Well, the team helps," he said. His group of riders had brought in $130,000 this year, pushing his ten-year fundraising total past the $425,000 mark. "That and corporate sponsorships. It's really important to get others involved and sell them on what you're doing. The more others can be connected and a part of it, the better."

I nodded. I needed to talk to more people or have others talk to more people on my behalf–or both, though it already felt like I was maxing out my network. Everyone I knew had already given.

We continued onward in a pack. The day's heat began to rise. As it had been recently, it would be stifling and sticky by noon.

"We're going to push on," Chuck's son said, indicating they'd like to pick up the pace. "Though Superman over here doesn't like to admit it, we need to get these miles done and over and get him into the shade as quickly as possible." Chuck had his limitations, after all, living with multiple sclerosis. MS didn't care if he was a state-winning quarterback or how much money he'd raised. Like my mother, it'd take what it would, and he'd have to manage what was left.

Chuck agreed. "Andy's right. But we'll see you at the VIP tent!" he said over his shoulder, already biking faster. "We'll save you a spot!"

And with that, my father and I were on our own.

Biking wasn't running, but I couldn't help but enjoy it too. It had a rhythm to it, much like running–different but repetitive all the same. I'd pedal hard up a hill and feel the metronome of my body working back and forth in unison with the bike. I'd glide down the other side and zone out to the *buzz* of the gears in a coast.

WORTH IT

The trees whipped past my body, and the air cooled my skin. I was free like I was in a run, but also, I wasn't stupid—at the turns, I'd squeeze the brakes tight and slow more than others, as any rational person who was biking 150 miles in the middle of running across America would. I was part riding the Tour de France and part conscious that a crash could sideline the thousand miles that remained to New York.

"So, Dad," I said later as we breezed along a lengthy stretch of soybeans. "What'd you think when I told you Nate proposed?"

He shrugged. "What do you mean? I knew about it before you did."

"You did?" I asked, surprised. All along, Nate's empty-handed-reaching-at-the-top-of-a-mountain-we-were-never-supposed-to-be-on proposal had given me the impression that it had been unplanned. Maybe I'd been wrong.

"Yup," my father said, his breathing was labored but far from capacity. "He asked me for your hand while we loaded up the RV. You were in the house, packing a few things."

"Really?"

"Yeah. It was kind of cute." My dad continued, "He was pretty nervous."

I thought of Nate being nervous about asking my dad if he could marry me, and I smiled. "What did he say to you? What did you say to him?"

"Well. He said, more or less, that he wanted to propose to you on a mountain, and would that be okay with me?"

"And what did you say to him?" I encouraged again before he could continue.

He looked my way and tilted his head. "He loves you. He cares about you. He came over here from Australia to help you run across America. I shook his hand and said yes. That your mom and I would be glad to have him in the family."

I nodded and smiled.

We rode on for a bit while I thought about the scene my father had described. Nate had planned the proposal—*and* he had also done as I'd asked, doing it without a ring because I'd insisted I didn't need one. He had also left his job and come over here from Australia, and he was the person helping me day after day while I ran across the country. Did his wanting to leave alter any of that? I wondered how love and care changed when things got difficult. I wondered what should be done when it does.

"How did you know you wanted to marry Mom?" I said after a while.

Before answering, he dropped his hand to the bike frame, took a swig from his water bottle, and then popped it back in its clip between his legs.

"You know," he said, "I could sit with her and just watch the grass grow. And that's all I needed to know. We didn't have to be doing anything in particular. I just liked being around her a whole lot. I still do."

He trained his gaze forward in the direction we were headed. "Life is like traveling in a canoe, and marriage is about picking who's in your boat. You want to make sure you enjoy the person, and it makes things a whole lot easier if you both paddle in the same direction."

I smiled at the thought. He made the complexities of picking a life partner as pleasant as a canoe trip. I didn't ask him, *How do you feel about caring for her? Do you ever want a break? Can you imagine wanting to leave her for a bit?*

Saying those things would give attention to thoughts I wished not to grow. And anyway, I already knew what he'd say. He had said it a million times over in the thirty-six years that they had been married. He'd never left her side.

Instead, I looked ahead too—and kept on pedaling.

We finally made it to the VIP tent well after lunch—with ten miles left in the day's ride, my knee felt sore, so I got a lift and waited for my father there. I found Chuck misting himself under a shaded pavilion, and I sat by his side while we cheered for the steady stream of riders coasting underneath a steel arch. A banner hung from its support beams—FINISH MS.

That evening, I sat next to my father at the rider's celebration dinner—a catered event hosted in a massive, white tent set up on the city's university park lawn, with circular tables and plastic folding chairs beneath. A stage at the front featured a giant projector screen and a singular microphone. Before it stood the chapter president.

"And together, this year, the ride has raised over"—she paused for effect—"$1.2 million to end MS!"

The crowd erupted in applause and cheers. The atmosphere shook with renewed hope.

One-point-two million dollars in one weekend, I thought. I had been on the road for months and had only raised $40,000 so far. It hardly seemed worth it when I weighed the effort against the result.

I could have done just as well by simply riding in this event.

As the president continued the program, calling the top fundraisers forward on stage—Chuck and other teams alike—my insides bubbled with envy. I heard the totals, hundreds of thousands of dollars each, and knew that I deserved to be up there as well, sharing my mother's story of joy and resilience, being honored with all the others for their immense impact on the cause.

But I couldn't deny that I actually *didn't*.

I had done an impressive amount of running and raised plenty of awareness, and that was about it. These people were taking only a weekend from their families and crushing my numbers fourfold.

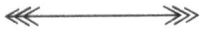

THREE DAYS LATER, I stood in the eastern parking lot of Miller Park, home of the Milwaukee Brewers baseball team. It was August 10, the day of my game-starting pitch, and I busied myself alongside Nate and my family, arranging the fundraising event space and hoping people would show.

We drove the motorhome from the hotel and parked it at the edge of the lot space, where we began to set up our merchandise table under its awning. A party tent big enough to hold a hundred people was being erected by Karl's Party Supply, adjacent to the RV, and next to that was Klement's Sausage Company, which had just arrived with three hundred brats, their grill, and a full-service concession table. I felt anxious at the sight of the Klement's crew, dressed in their linen chef aprons, laying out hundreds of links in shiny aluminum pans. I tugged at the bottom of my canvas shorts again, adjusting my clothes the way I wished to adjust my anxiety, and with that, my stomach fluttered. I felt as if I were standing upon a towering bridge, preparing for a bungee jump. Three hundred was *a lot* of sausages.

"Ashley!"

Someone had shouted my name. I turned, and across the open asphalt in the bright sun was a friend from high school with her parents.

"Hollie!" I shouted back.

"Ashley," they said again, finally arriving at the motorhome with open arms.

I moved forward to hug each—Hollie first, a long, tight embrace, then her mother, then her father. Hollie and I had been inseparable during high school. It felt good to see familiar faces.

"I can hardly believe it," her mother said. "You are running across America."

"I know," I said with wide eyes.

"Are you kidding me?" her father said. "This girl ran everywhere in high school. You were made for this."

"I know," I said again with wide eyes, and we all laughed.

"So, what? Everything's great? Your body is good? I need you to update that blog more. I'm on edge each day waiting for updates," her mother said.

"I know. I know. I mean to blog more. I just…" I shook my head. "The days go by faster than I imagined."

"Leave her be, Mom," Hollie said, wrapping both her arms around my body, giving me a squeeze. "She's doing great! Plus, more importantly, where's this Australian fiancé of yours?"

Just then, Nate opened the entry door from the motorhome, bounding down the steps from where he'd been sitting with my mother inside. She'd been cooling herself in the air conditioning.

I introduced him to Hollie and her parents, then got the family settled at the merchandise table where they planned to volunteer to manage the money—T-shirt purchases, brat sales, and donations.

Folding the merchandise T-shirts, I wiped another bead of sweat from my brow. Nearing the noon hour, the day's temperatures were rising to an intense and sticky eighty-four degrees. Something about standing in an asphalt parking lot on a breezeless August day made me realize how much people would need the party tent.

"AK!" a friend from college shouted. She walked to me with others from the soccer team, all of them in town from out of state, specifically for this fundraising event.

"You ran here, you crazy fool!" one of them joked. "Next time, just take a plane."

"I know, right?" I said, giving her and the others a hug.

We caught up, talking about my run and reminiscing about time together on the soccer pitch. They joked about how absurd I had been back then, and their candor brought me ease. I wasn't a nonprofit founder fumbling over fundraising. I wasn't a runner they saw each week on Fox Sports, though I was. I was AK–a girl they knew well from years of playing soccer together and too many drunken nights to count.

Just then, Dawn came into the circle.

"Hey," she said, breathless from a quick run across the event space. "Montel is here."

"Oh." I clapped, glancing at my friends. "I must go now. I am very important."

They each gave me a look, and Steph, my closest friend, rolled her eyes.

"Okay, but really, the brats are over there, seats over here, merch behind me, and the Racing Sausages should be here in an hour," I said, talking toward them while walking away with Dawn.

The next hour and a half melted away in this manner—me in a conversation with someone I hadn't seen in months or years, and then someone or something else calling for my attention. Nate mingled about too, appearing in good spirits when I took care to look his way. He caught up with the reporter doing weekly broadcasts of my run. He laughed with my father about something I couldn't hear. He stood smiling next to a giant sausage mascot for a photo. He encouraged everyone to go to the merchandise table and buy a shirt—replicas of the very one he wore. I watched him, glad that he was finally having a good time. If I hadn't been at his side when he'd called his role "mundane," I may not have believed it happened.

Finally, the start of the game neared, made evident by the Brewers staffer who drove the quarter mile from the stadium into our tailgate event in a shuttle golf cart.

"You ready?" she asked, which was more of a statement than a question, so I gathered up my parents and climbed aboard—them in the second row behind her and Dawn and me on the back. Nate hitched a ride on another golf cart with Montel and his wife.

Zipping toward the building, we passed groups of people doing what I had—chugging beer, flipping red Solo cups on a table, and screaming loudly at each other in laughter. It wasn't that long ago that baseball games had been yet another excuse for me to binge drink and feel normal about it. Someone would buy a pack of tickets, and one way or another, a ticket would make its way to me.

Brewers games meant grilling, bags, flip cup, and a line of coolers across three parking spaces full of ice and alcohol. Beer in this one, rum in that one, mixers over there, and a Bloody Mary bar here if you're still hung over from the day before. It was drink as much as you could before you went inside because beer inside was twelve bucks. It was, *Fuck it. I don't care that the beer is twelve bucks. This is great. Everyone, get a round. Here's my card.* It was one round turning into many, turning into puke splattered across a bathroom stall. It was a hot dog and fries afterward because shit food soaks up alcohol.

I passed the crowds riding in a golf cart and felt a nostalgic pull for those carefree, booze-filled days. It was the fun and freedom that I missed, and I regularly wondered about how the nonprofit would change that for me. Still, I wanted what lay ahead of me.

Back toward the south side of the stadium, the staffer drove us to a barricaded loading area at a tunnel leading underneath the building. She drove into the opening, and the sunlight shrank behind us. A line of fluorescent lights illuminated walls of cool, gray concrete. At an unmarked door—an opening much larger than a regular door—the golf cart came to a stop.

"Okay," she said. "We'll just wait here for a bit." Then she picked up her smartphone and started pecking away.

My mom leaned toward my father. "Where's Montel?"

"Around here somewhere, I'm sure," my dad replied.

"I want to show him my poems," she said in return, looking straight ahead at the doors. "Maybe he can read them on TV."

Without a word, my father gently patted her leg.

Did I want my mother to corner Montel at my cross-country charity event when it was a miracle he was here in the first place, supporting it and generating sponsors to pay for it? Not exactly. But I didn't not want her to either. In a world that could beat you out of your dreams with its sensibility, I couldn't help but find her motives endearing. Despite it all, her dreams remained. I took note. I always had.

"And now, back in her hometown of Milwaukee, Wisconsin, after running all the way here from California—Ashley Kumlien of MS Run the US, here to throw out the first pitch!"

The oversized door we'd parked at opened inward toward me, and I ran through the opening into the stadium.

Relax your shoulders. Smile. Just run. I coached myself, hoping not to trip.

My parents and Dawn had already been whisked away down the long concrete hallway toward the Brewers' dugout.

"Wait here," the staffer had said. "When this door opens, run through it and head down the warning track toward home plate. When you're even with the pitcher's mound, cut across the grass to meet your mom. Your sister will be there with her. Stay off the outfield grass, okay?"

"Okay," I said.

Then she climbed onto the golf cart and left me by myself next to the oversized door. With them gone, I noticed a line of industrial rugs that lay across the polished floor in sections. I wiggled my foot on the bare floor surface beneath me and heard the squeak echo off the empty hallway while I waited.

That I was standing in the Brewers' private staging area waiting to run in front of thirty-five thousand fans and throw out the game's first pitch didn't faze me. Like the first day of my run at the Golden Gate Bridge, I remained steady. The door would open, as doors do, and I would run. I wouldn't wave exuberantly and look about cheering like a person who couldn't contain themself—I'd keep my eyes forward, and I'd smile.

I'd run down the warning track and, at the designated spot as the staffer had asked, I'd cut across the infield toward the pitcher's mound. I'd meet my mother, where Nate and Dawn stood at her sides, and from her palm, I'd take a baseball. I'd kiss her cheek and turn toward home plate. I'd pull my arm back and, as I knew I would, throw the ball directly at the catcher. A tiny part of me that I kept contained would be relieved.

Afterward, I stood in front of a camera and a blaze of light next to a sideline reporter.

"Before you run away from us again," he said, "what can you tell us about your motivation to run across America?"

He held a microphone with a fluffy foam top toward my face.

"This is my mom," I said, tucking my arm into hers. She stood at my side with Dawn's help. Behind her was Nate, and on the other side of the reporter was Montel Williams. Out of view, happily avoiding interview questions, was my father.

"She was diagnosed with multiple sclerosis before I was born. I'm running to help fund MS research."

"And is it correct," the reporter said, looking at his cue card, "that you had never run a marathon before deciding to do this?"

"Yes, that's true." I blushed.

"And you're perfectly healthy? Having run"—he looked at his card again—"2,388 miles in four months to get here?"

"So far, so good," I said, smiling.

He shook his head. "Incredible. Now, Montel, you live with MS yourself. What do you want people to know about MS?"

"You know, I was told I'd be in a wheelchair by now," Montel started. "That's what doctors say to people diagnosed with MS. They give them a death sentence. But I'm not. I'm standing next to you, and standing by that amazing woman over there running all the way across this country to raise awareness for this horrible disease, because I took the time to change my diet and my lifestyle to fight the debilitating effects it has on the body. And I'm one of the lucky ones."

"So they gave you a death sentence?" the reporter repeated.

"That's what it felt like," Montel said. "That's what someone hears when you're healthy and walking, and then are told you have MS and will end up in a wheelchair. It changes your whole life. But because of people like Ashley, out here raising money, every single day, there's a breakthrough coming with MS. Ten years ago, when you said MS, no one knew what this was. Now, what everyone needs to understand is that everyone listening right now has someone in their family or someone they know who is touched by this disease, and it's people like Ashley who are raising money who give us all hope."

"It's an amazing effort," the reporter said. "And I am excited to say that the Brewers' Community Foundation believes in what you're doing."

Just then, the director of the foundation walked toward us with one of those giant checks. The words "MS RUN THE US" were printed across the top with an amount of $2,500 written in the monetary box. I heard Dawn sob.

Forty-two thousand dollars, I said to myself, adding it to my overall total.

It wasn't enough.

I was grateful, but still, it wasn't enough.

I grabbed a corner of the stiff plastic board and smiled for photos. Later, I would awkwardly make my way out of the stadium with it stuffed under my arm like a human billboard. At my parents' house, I'd tip it up on its side and tuck it between the wall and my desk. Where else does someone stow a giant check? Sometime later, I'd pull it back out, adding more zeros to it with a permanent marker, if for no other reason than simply to imagine what it would feel like to truly make a difference.

"I'm impressed," Steph said at my side after the check presentation. It was the fifth inning, and we were milling about in the box suite that the Brewers had provided. In it, we had been joined by

Nate, my family, Montel and his wife, and a small cluster of media executives.

"I was a little worried you weren't going to make the plate," she joked.

"I'm just really talented," I said to her sarcastically.

She laughed. "You're dumb."

I smiled.

"So, the blogs have been interesting. You want to talk about it or not really?" she asked.

I tilted my head side to side. In addition to the elusive blog I'd written about my fight with Nate, he wanted to write one of his own, sharing his view—from the driver's side, he called it—and then compared helping me to the same as watching 540 hours of tennis, which would "definitely get boring, even for the ultimate tennis fan."

"I mean, I get it," I started, digging my finger into my nail bed. "He's basically sitting out on the highway for hours while I run. He's not making any money, and he's really far away from home. So I think the whole thing is just different than we'd thought. He's going to take a break at my parents' place for the next couple weeks while they come out and crew me."

"You mentioned that on the phone," she said.

Braun hit a double. The stadium erupted.

"But, you know," she continued after the cheering subsided, "he did sign up for this. He volunteered to come with you. He told you he wanted to. You didn't force him to do this."

I looked at her, and she stared right back at me. Across the room, Nate made a gesture with his hand to the group he was with. Everyone laughed.

"I know," I said to Steph. "It's just complicated. Is it the event? Is this us? I'm just not sure." I took a drink from the beer in my hand. Its chilled aluminum surface cooled the tips of my fingers.

"Hey," she said, touching my arm. "I'm proud of you. What you're doing is big. I've watched you today and listened to how you respond to praise. You're normalizing this, and it's not normal. People don't do what you're doing—they don't quit their jobs, build a charity, and run thousands of miles for their mom. You have a gift, and you're using it to make a difference. That's unique. Don't forget that while you're out there on the road by yourself, wondering if you're worth being cared for. Okay?"

Tears welled in my eyes. I looked away from her toward the baseball field, waiting until I was sure the tears wouldn't spill over.

"Okay," I said, watching the pitcher rocket the ball over home plate.

Then I looked at her and nodded. "Okay."

PART 3
Searching Middle

CHAPTER TWENTY

Crossroads

"THE WIPES ARE IN that bag," said my father, pointing to a stiff polyester US Bank duffel bag in the corner—a freebie for those who could be baited into opening a new account for such things. My father was this kind of person.

My mother was motionless on her back across the RV's queen bed while my father shimmied a pair of soiled Depends down her porcelain, chalky legs. Her elastic waistband pants were on the floor, soaked through, and all she could do was lie there, vacant in body but fully present in mind. My dad moved around her idle limbs in an experienced frenzy. The desperate, longing look in her eyes prickled the skin on the back of my neck.

It was just before six in the morning. We were somewhere in Ohio, and today was a bad MS day.

Her physical being, limbs, and larynx were immobile, yet she was there—aware of her paralysis and unable to do anything about it. I could turn from it if I wanted to, as I had been doing until recently, but that wouldn't change what was—there's no outrunning MS, if that's what's coming for you.

I bent down now to open the flap of the US Bank duffel bag to retrieve what my father had asked for. The wipe's flimsy plastic bag crinkled in my hands. My father moved now in a way that told me this experience wasn't new to him—that he had done this before within the comforts of their own home, the very walls in which I grew. They would be there now if Nate hadn't needed to rest.

The only thing new here was me.

"Could you grab a clean pair of pants?" my father directed. "And the Depends are in a bag in the closet."

I moved with a gentle purpose. His desire, I knew, was to do this alone—to be in the privacy of his own home watching after his wife in all the ways required of a caregiver that nobody liked to think about, like wiggling disposable underwear off their bodies and wiping limp limbs clean of waste.

He worked on removing the Depends now as efficiently as possible and then cleaned her over and over again with wipes meant for babies. He touched his hand on her thigh, on her arm, on her calf as he wiped, signaling to her that he was there, always in contact. Together, we shimmied into a clean pair of the disposable underwear and elastic band jeans before propping her comfortably onto pillows.

I checked my phone for the time. It was 6:33 a.m.

And this, I thought, *is why they never visited me on ships.*

Oh, how I'd begged my dad to book a cruise with her when I'd worked at sea.

"There's a family discount," I'd coaxed. "I'll get you and Mom the best suite! And then, when we get to St. John, you can go scuba diving while I stay with her! Please? You haven't been diving in how long?"

The answer was forever. He hadn't been diving in forever. It was something he had done in his youth—before kids, before the diagnosis, while he and Mom had still been dating. He'd pack up his two-door Duster and head to Florida with his brother to dive with the barracudas. But he hadn't made time since. His wetsuit hung in the laundry room at home, a hollow form of the life he'd once lived.

"Meister," he'd reply. "I just... I don't want to go where she can't."

Where she can't, I assumed, meant that he didn't want to go diving if she couldn't.

What's the big deal? I thought. *Why not?*

But now I swallowed the truth like rocks. He wasn't thinking about grand adventures under the water's surface to explore the ocean floor. He was nowhere near that experience. He lived in a far less grand place–underwater in a whole different sense, thinking not of Caribbean ports, but rather, the anxiety of being at sea with his wife, who could need advanced medical care at any moment– and the astronomical cost they'd pay if she had to be flown to the nearest land hospital.

I'd thought he'd lacked the ambition to visit me, when actually he'd been protecting me from a harsh truth that, I'll admit, I hadn't wanted to know–that their reality was far more difficult than I'd imagined.

They awoke each day to the possibility of daunting tasks, like wiping a body as cooperative as a hundred-pound bag of Jell-O clean of waste. And yet, they went on. Whether they awoke to this or dodged it altogether and went straight for coffee, I would have never known. He'd never told me that days like this had been happening for years. Why would he? What good would come of it?

In time, he'd let go of his adventures and embraced the view from his front porch. After what I'd just experienced with them, I'd be content with that as well.

I had left Wisconsin the day after my pitch at the Brewers' game with my parents in tow, to crew me through what remained of Illinois, all of Indiana, and part of Ohio. With them by my side and Nate resting at their house, days became fluid.

"How's 4:45 a.m. for you?" I asked tentatively about the morning alarm I'd set for our first night staying together in the RV. They'd sleep in the queen bed in back while I'd take the futon couch across from the entry door. We were at a campground in Illinois, just an hour away from the border of Indiana.

"Fine with us." My father shrugged.

When that time came the next morning, they were already awake, waiting for me.

Each evening thereafter, I kissed them goodnight, laid out my clothes and phone on the dinette seat across from where I slept, and fell fast asleep. Come morning, with a warm splash of water on the face and a handful of grapes for breakfast, my parents were ready to go almost as quickly as I could brush my teeth and get dressed. My father would pour their coffee into to-go mugs, add cream and sugar, and then set them in the car's cupholders before he and I would assist my mother down the four steep motorhome steps—me in the front to steady her while my father held on tight from the back.

This space, of course, was more cumbersome than what we all were used to—me with Nate not needing my help to move around, and them having already worked out maneuvering techniques at home. Still, their cheerfulness made everything seem okay. Even showering my mother every few days—slowly walking her to the campground's shower house, sitting her on the metal and cloth camp chair that we used as a disability shower seat, bathing her and redressing her after having already run a marathon myself for the day—felt doable. She was happy to be adventuring with me, and I was glad to have them along—them being upbeat and optimistic about each day.

And with these experiences, I could no longer deny that I had become emotionally exhausted prior to Milwaukee. That all my running around to make pesky tasks seem like no problem at all was all quite tiring.

Now, my days passed with ease. I *enjoyed* running across the Illinois border and then across the whole state of Indiana. I danced at the state line while my mother cheered from the car. My father, of course, filled our days with interesting facts—something he had been doing all along via email, yet now he simply told me in person.

"General 'Mad' Anthony Wayne," he'd say into the silence while I ate a banana at the car during a crew stop. "That's where Fort Wayne got its name. It held a key position in the Pennsylvania Railroad because of the three rivers here." He gazed across the moving river just beyond the car, imagining it now.

I ran, my mother encouraged, and he'd recite what he'd read from whatever place he'd read it—sometimes from a historical marker, other times from an internet search. Indiana was the

CROSSROADS

"Crossroads of America," he told me. It was the state's motto—a fact that, later, had me thinking about the irony of it.

I was at a crossroads myself.

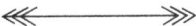

"OKAY, YOU'RE GOOD FOR a bit?" my father asked as he pulled the car over on a side street somewhere in Ohio, just north of Columbus. We had gotten my mom changed and settled, grabbed a quick bite, and then went out the door so I could run twenty-six miles.

"Yup. I have my hydration pack and some bars. I'll be good for at least three hours," I told him with confidence. "Plus, I have my phone and some money. I'll call you if I need you."

"Check in every hour," he reminded me before I shut the door. I smiled and waved in response. Of being self-reliant, I was well equipped for this role—having run here from San Francisco, having worked at needing no one.

He waved and drove away in the direction that we'd come.

Standing on the side of the road, I watched their Chevy disappear—the same car that had crewed me through my first impromptu marathon, through my first fifty-mile race, and through the ambitious events thereafter, to here, where I turned from it and ran east on a highway toward New York.

Making my way out of the tiny town, a place called Pharisburg, I came to Highway 37 and continued on. Narrowing roads in the east had the cars whipping past my body like earthbound rockets, and yet, the therapy of running lulled me into an ease. My shoulders, bound from bending and lifting my mother, loosened. The sound of my feet upon pavement, a trustworthy beat. My lungs breathed a steady flow. It was a chorus of sameness, and it comforted me.

Running along, I kept my gaze ahead at a bright horizon that met the road that I ran—a charcoal-gray path striped with its yellow and white rules.

If only life were that simple, I thought.

That if you stayed within the lines, then no one would get hurt.

I couldn't help but let my mind wander to Nate, as it had been since I'd last seen him weeks ago. He'd stayed back, able-bodied but needing a break, while my burdened parents had taken his place.

He slept in while we cleaned shit from skin—a thought that came so abruptly to my mind that a suffering, sad sob erupted from within and heaved me forward, as if I had been punched in the gut. The injustice of her disease, the lack of funds I was raising, and the man who I loved being unable to do this work all toppled over until the mass of pain I'd fought to subdue broke free of its reins, and I cried.

The temperature rose. An hour passed, and then another. I was running again after gasping for air through the hard, awful tears that had come. They'd landed safely, in a soft, solitary space. When they were through, I had stood, seeing my sun-cast shadow stretch out along the pavement—my reflection standing tall with me. A light breeze had come upon my hot, damp skin. Stalks of corn had stretched toward the sun, swaying gently.

I sighed a deep breath. Running met me where I was, like a reliable friend, and melted my heartache like the ice in my pack. Moving along, sweat pooled thick on my skin. The sun, now high into the sky, baked the highway and its roadkill into a scented array of rubber and bloated death. Flies swarmed, feasting and laying maggots, and I ran past holding my breath. It was the dead of summer, and I was roasting, but on I went, wishing not to be anywhere else. I'd run this highway forever if it meant that I could.

Sometime later, I slowed to a walk and called my father after squeezing the last of my melted gummies into my mouth. This route would take me through places called Sunbury, Mt. Vernon, Sugarcreek, and Carrollton before I'd run out of Ohio, seven days from now, along a beautiful, winding river near East Steubenville. For now, though, I was simply twenty-four miles east of where he'd last seen me.

"Hey, Dad. How's Mom?" I asked on the phone.

"She's sleeping," he replied. "I cranked up the AC, and I think it's doing her some good. How about you?"

"Not bad," I told him. I swallowed the glob of sugar, and my tummy let out an audible rumble. "I could eat. You think you can come grab me soon? Otherwise, I'll figure out what's ahead and manage for a bit."

"She's in a good spot," he told me. "I'll hop in the car now."

I walked a tight space between the ditch and traffic until he came upon me and pulled off the road into a plot of grass just ahead. The generous shoulders I'd run on throughout Indiana—happy spaces, sometimes the width of a car—were gone. Now, hurried trucks just feet from my reach drove along paved paths not accustomed to pedestrians—the cars' lack of braking and their drivers' honking told me so.

"I passed a Subway in Delaware," I said, opening the passenger door to my father's vehicle. "You think we can grab a few subs before heading back?"

"Yeah, that'll be good," he replied. "Get something with bacon for your mother, and I'll take the roasted chicken." He handed me his credit card from his wallet, a rubber band wrapped twice around a stack of cards and cash. He pulled the car back onto the highway. A short time later, he saw something he couldn't pass up.

"Oh, even better!" he exclaimed.

"We're going to stop, aren't we?" I joked.

"You bet." He smiled. "There's a banana and cookie in that bag. I figured you might be hungry."

Standing in front of the historical marker of Major General William Starke Rosecrans, I became absorbed. His bronzed horse-mounted figure stood upon a forty-thousand-pound boulder pushed here by Wisconsin glaciers over 180,000 years ago. I put my fingers upon its rough surface, and it, too, like me, felt scorched by the sun. The major sat on his horse with a buckaroo hat upon his head and a sword in its sheath like a man on top of the world. He'd been a soldier, an engineer, an architect, and an inventor. He'd been an integral part of development in this region, and the man had raised $789,000 for soldier relief in the mid-1800s. My run now, 168 years after his efforts, crawled toward the $50,000 mark.

How did he do it? I wondered.

"Did you see about the boulder?" My dad said, interrupting my thoughts. "It traveled here from Wisconsin, just like you."

"I did," I said, smiling at the thought. "Did you see about Mr. Major General here?"

"I did." He nodded. "Sounds like a busy guy."

He was well accomplished. I wanted to be a busy guy.

"Should we get back to Mom?" I asked.

"Sure."

We started toward the car.

"She'll be okay, kid," he said, sensing my mood–a weightedness that accompanied me now after the morning's events, after running myself dry of tears. "She just has to sleep it off."

"I know," I replied. "It just sucks."

"I get it, but listen." He stopped walking. "We're doing okay. That's not something I hoped you'd be part of, but we're doing okay. Your mom and I always remind each other that if we got together with a bunch of people and threw our problems into a pile, we'd go ahead and grab our own problems right back."

"I know," I admitted, knowing it was true. "You're right."

I looked down at the colonial brick path beneath my feet. It was immaculate and level in every way, except for a few tiny blades of grass breaking through the cracks. They were little shoots of life living above the weight.

Somehow, my father always knew exactly what to say, though it didn't fully ease what was building within me. Their time on the road was coming to an end, and I'd rather they stayed. It wasn't just the morning. It was all of it.

"There's other stuff, too, you know," I said, standing at his side. "Nate. The fundraising. All the things I thought this would be. I've never felt so confused about what I should be doing. It's a lot all at once."

He stood for a bit before saying anything. "It's hard to know how it's all going to go. Sometimes you just have to wait it out. When your mom was diagnosed, we never could have known that we'd have you, and that you'd do this. We just picked ourselves up and took it one day at a time. We've had some good days and some really hard days, but you running across America for her has brought a new meaning to it all. It took some time, but here we are."

"*Some time?* That was like thirty years ago!" I blurted out. "I'll *die* if I have to wait that long to figure this out."

"Oh, come on," he said lightly. "We can laugh about it, or we can cry about it. And laughing is a lot more fun. Okay? Who knows–you could get a big donation any day now! Oprah could be watching."

"Oh, God. Oprah," I said. "Then Mom would die."

He laughed, and I couldn't help but join him. Then he wrapped his arms around me, and I squeezed him back, tight.

I breathed him in–his Old Spice aftershave, his worn cotton T-shirt, the firmness of his pot belly. Turning to walk again, I missed them terribly already. Of all the things I relied on myself for, I could always depend on them for this–my parents never let me stay down.

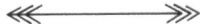

FOUR DAYS LATER, IN central Ohio, my friend, Dan, from Milwaukee, drove the charity's vehicle into Timbercrest campground just before dinner time. Even at a crawling speed–five miles per hour, per the campground rules–the parched gravel kicked up a plume of dust in Dan's wake.

The place was a treeless field of grass cut into gravel lots with water spigots raised from the ground like tiny flag poles. It wasn't notable–not a place I'd pick to dazzle anyone new into the RV life. Rather, when it came time to set up camp the day prior, my parents and I had picked it because it met my only two requirements–that it had a handicap shower stall for my mother, and that it was minutes from my route, where I had been weaving myself through Ohio along the quiet Amish country side, mostly undisturbed except for the occasional *clopping* of horseshoes on asphalt, pulling a single carriage buggy.

The occupants would pass, and I'd take in their wide-brimmed hats and orange hazard triangle. I'd wonder about their unusual life. I'd wonder if they wondered about mine. Then I'd finish for the day and wish to be as close to the camper as possible–to shower, to eat, to collapse my body onto a stretch of blankets in

THE LONG RUN HOME

the air conditioning and take a nap. So really, it didn't matter if the campsite was a resort or otherwise.

The car came to a stop at our barren site, covered it in a thin layer of chalky powder, and with it, Nate—the passenger, along with Dan—was back.

"Hey!" I greeted him, bounding out of the RV with the same enthusiasm I poured into our texts and playful banter.

"Babe!" he exclaimed, his arms open wide, walking toward me. I went to him and threw my arms around his neck. He picked me up in a tight squeeze.

"I missed you!" he said. "I missed this orange bus!"

My heart jumped. Did he mean it?

He set me down, and we kissed—though rather quickly with Dan now out of the car and at our side. "Almost to Pennsylvania! You guys ready for this?"

"Oh man! I can't wait!" Dan said, beaming with a natural intensity that put toddlers to shame. "When do we run next?"

"I'm done for the day, and it's hot as hell. But if you need to move, I can show you where to run," I told him.

Dan was the type who needed to move. We'd met at an ultramarathon race the year prior and had continued a friendship over our shared interest in charity work and running farther than people thought reasonable to do. He was lean in the way one would imagine an ultra runner to be (though I had seen my fair share of other types) and had buzz-cut hair atop the face of a baby. His plethora of energy needed a place to go. Running for twenty-four hours to see how far he could get often did the trick.

"Oh man! That would be great!" he said, bouncing in place. "That eight-hour drive from Wisconsin was brutal."

"You got it," I said, clapping him on the shoulder. "How about you guys get settled while I say goodbye to my parents? Then we'll look at the map."

He and Nate moved toward the car to get their bags. Already, Dan was the buffer that Nate and I needed to continue ignoring the feelings that had erupted in Iowa.

I hadn't faked my excitement just now, or even the banter between us during the weeks we spent apart, just to lure him back to the road. I was earnestly trying. I knew why I loved him and remembered why he was out here in the first place—all the dreams we'd dreamed together lying across a deck chair on the fourteenth floor of a cruise ship.

But now everything felt murky—the space between us muddied by the challenges of the road and his attempt to dodge them. The morning that my mother awoke immobile five days ago, which I'd never told him about, only widened the gap. I couldn't imagine getting the words out without him feeling like, in part, he was at fault, with them being here because he chose not to be.

I wasn't sure if I thought he wasn't.

What did he know of having to shower his mother or wipe her clean? From what I knew, his was in Australia living just minutes from the ocean in a spotless house with a backyard pool and a parakeet named Jacko. Could he understand these complex feelings if I tried to explain them? But also, he'd met my mother and experienced my father's hoarding. What was there to explain?

What was building at the time was something I only came to understand much later as a complicated, multi-layered emotion called resentment. I was twenty-eight days from my finish in New York, with the tasks that drove him to stay back still plentiful ahead of us. If he truly missed it, I would know soon enough.

"All set?" I called out to my father, who was loading up their car to leave. It was late in the day, but he was a seasoned driver. He'd make the full eight-hour drive back to Wisconsin just fine, only stopping if my mom had to use the bathroom.

"I think so," my dad replied, closing the trunk with a thud. The license plate rattled.

"You need me to take her to the bathroom?" I offered. My mom sat patiently in the passenger seat.

"Nah, I haven't given her fluids since lunch, and I made her go before putting her in the car."

"All right then," I said lightly. "Thanks for coming. Drive safe. See you in New York. All that kind of stuff."

Laugh about it or cry about it, he had said. I was determined not to cry.

"Here," he said, handing me an unused Subway napkin with his all-capitalized penmanship across the back. Both were trademarks of my father—the writing of things on napkins and every letter in its parent form. On it was the title of a poem he and I had shared throughout the years. It said DON'T QUIT—J. WHITTIER.

I looked at the translucent paper and said nothing at first, thumbing its textured corner. The poem was about forging on when life gets you down. I had used it in high school as encouragement for hard tests or cross-country races or when it got back to me that So-and-So had said such-and-such about me to someone who mattered, which all seemed so silly now that I thought about my father using it to pull himself out of bed and into a full day of work while caring for my mother and their four children. He was so much more resolute than I'd ever given him credit for.

"Thanks, Dad," I said finally, giving him a squeeze.

He'd say nothing else, him being a man of few words, and us having already said what needed to be said.

Moving to the car, I gave my mom a hug too, leaning down through the open door and putting my arms around her as best as I could.

"I'll see you in New York," I told her with a smile.

"See you in New York." She smiled back.

It wasn't until their car had disappeared and the gravel dust settled that I considered the poem again, the flimsy note still weightless in my hand.

Don't quit, he'd encouraged.

As I stood there thinking about it, I couldn't be certain what he hoped I'd endure.

Was it the fundraising?

Or the relationship?

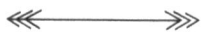

THE NEXT MORNING, I slept in, easing into what would be a scorching September day. With Nate back, I interrupted my pre-dawn wake-up regimen for the moment, hoping to gently bring him back to the road. And, if I'm being honest, it was nice to cozy up next to him again. We had slept through the night with our limbs entangled, us together on the queen bed in back while Dan took the futon couch up front.

The midmorning light shone through closed window shades, and I saw his chocolate-brown eyes open.

"How'd you sleep?" I asked him quietly after a moment, his face just inches from mine.

"Good," he whispered back. "It's like I never left."

I smiled.

He stretched, arching his back, reaching his arms, sighing.

"So, what are you thinking?" I asked. "You want to run with me this morning?"

"Yeah, let's do it," he replied, yawning.

One of the benefits of having Dan on the road with us now, a second crew person, was that each could swap out driving and running. No one person was confined to the car for the entire day. Nate could run while Dan drove, and then Dan could run while Nate drove. We'd share cooking, shopping, cleanup, and nearly every other task except for camp setup and takedown, which was simple enough but not worth a full tutorial with Dan only around for the week. Dan was also chatty and rather outgoing, a welcome reprieve for Nate, I imagined, in comparison to my more internal ways. I couldn't help but notice that a jolt of life had returned to his energy.

"You up, mate?" Nate called out softly to the living area.

"Yeah, I'm up," Dan replied. "Let's get this party started!"

Running the increasing and undulating hills of eastern Ohio *was* a party for Dan, and thanks to the 2,700 miles I ran to get there and the miracle that was my body's ability to do it, it was a party for me too. I hadn't deteriorated, as many had worried I would. My tendons didn't ache with inflammation. My bones didn't fracture under the stress. Rather, I was just fine. My body was lean and efficient, my legs tanned and strong. I tied on my shoes each morning and ran, mile upon mile, for at least twenty-six miles, often more, and then afterward rolled right into the various tasks that needed to be done as I neared my anticipated finish. Dan and I ran side by side, discussing these things along a highway shaded in a canopy of towering oak trees, some days after his arrival.

"I have to admit, this is harder than I expected it to be," Dan said after cresting another hill.

"What? The hills?" I asked, my breath labored but controlled.

"That," he replied. "And all of it." He stopped talking for a few breaths. "Watching from home, it's easy to imagine that it's just running for five hours, and then the rest of the day is lounging around and recovering." He paused for a few moments again. "But there's a lot that goes into the pre-run and post-run that's hard to know unless you're here to witness it. Plus, all the messaging you do for the fundraising. You really never stop."

"Uh-huh," I agreed. "Nate and I have both tried to share what it's like, but it's not easy to explain."

"Like, I'm not sure people know how much time you spend preparing food and eating it," Dan said with a chuckle. "I bet you eat just as much as you run."

A laugh burst from within. I did spend a lot of time eating, having a meal or snack almost every hour that I wasn't running or sleeping.

"I have to. It keeps me going," I said. " I've already lost all the weight I gained from before the start and then some. I really can't stand to lose any more."

Dan and I let our legs cycle, coasting toward the base of a long decline. Today was his fourth day on the road with Nate and me, and everyone, including me, was feeling a touch sore from the up and down elevation. We were nearing the Appalachians, and with both Nate and Dan rotating through miles with me, I ran faster and longer than I would have alone.

"Did you send that email out about fundraising?" he asked, mentioning a conversation we'd had over a plate of chicken and rice the night before—about the astronomical amount of money I had left to raise before reaching my half-million-dollar goal.

"I did," I replied. It was another plea to the same pool of people who had already donated and supported my journey—to share with their friends and family. "I saw a few donations come in," I said. "But not what's needed, ya know?"

As we emerged from the canopy, the highway was hugged tight by a galvanized guardrail edging the space between a long, sloping embankment and the highway. Dan and I moved into single file form until a truck appeared from around the bend ahead. He and I hopped over the guardrail, standing on a slender patch of land. Then we jumped back over after the truck had *whooshed* past our noses.

"What if I write up a blog for you—to try to help explain how things are and why you're out here?" he offered. "Maybe it'll give your readers and my audience a different perspective? Would that help?"

"I can't see why not!" I said, excited and willing to try anything. The time I spent blogging and the desire to do so had drastically declined since Iowa. What was the point of making this seem like something it wasn't—pretending that everything was figured out? I couldn't. But maybe Dan could help. Maybe he'd write something the masses thought worth reading.

Just up the highway, we spotted the car pulled off onto a flat patch of grass. Nate stood near the trunk with a camera to his face, taking pictures of Dan and me coming up the narrow path.

"Eleven miles," Nate said of the distance we had just covered. "You ready to swap?" he asked Dan.

"You bet, man!" Dan said, happy to do almost anything. "My glutes are on fire from these hills!"

"Me too, mate. Running out here is no joke."

"Yeah. Ya know, it's one of the things I *love* about this whole thing," Dan said, emphasizing the word *love*. He stood at the trunk, digging through a plethora of food supplies, looking until he found an orange. "It's like, we're so capable, you know? But not many people even think to run this far. And then Ashley comes along and just *decides* to do this, and then *actually* does it." He tossed a chunk of peel into a plastic bag and then tapped his sweat-sheened forehead with his fingers. "It's all up here, ya know?"

"Yeah, mate," Nate said. "For sure."

We stood there for a bit, eating crunchy chips and oranges dripping with juice, listening to Dan speak passionately about the shortcomings of our culture. His personal story was one of drastic transformation, of following a traditional path through doctoral school, and then leaving it all behind after a visit to Thailand to spread a more altruistic message of unattached giving. It made having him easy. He never needed more than to simply be fed. He was intelligent and entertaining, if not a bit whimsical.

A tanker passed by, blaring its horn.

"Let's get off this thing," Nate said, looking around. "There's gotta be a back highway we can take."

I shook my head. "We kind of already passed it. There was a small road a couple miles back that cut through, but even then, we still have to cross into Pennsylvania through West Virginia and run Highway 22 for a bit. It'd give us a mile of peace. Maybe two." I shrugged. It just was what it was—there was no easy way about the route now. The topography thrust and bent as we neared the Appalachian range, making corners tight and vehicles close. There was no safer path than the one we were on because, simply, there was no safe path.

"It's not that bad," Dan encouraged. "I've been waving my arms, and people have been good about getting out of the way—even if they do like using their horns."

Nate nodded, seeming to understand we had limited options. "All right then," he said, bending down to tighten his laces and then standing to take off his shirt. "You ready, babe?"

"Let's do it," I said, eager to keep moving.

We ran for a bit, falling into the rhythm of moving as a pair, and then single file when the road called for it. I was proud of Nate covering the miles he had been recently. Not being one to find great pleasure in running, logging eleven miles at my side was something worth noting.

Being with Nate now was a mix of knowing what to say and not knowing exactly what not to say. There were the things we could talk about with ease—what he'd done with his days while he'd rested at my parents' place, when he'd last messaged his brother, what day and location would be the best for him to fly home from, how excited he was.

And then, there were the precarious topics that needed to be discussed at some point—where and when we should get married (now that he'd overstayed his vacation visa and would be denied another) and how we would pay for it, where would we live and how we would pay for it, who would take the charity across America again and how we would pay for it. *We'll figure it out* no longer seemed to suffice. He stopped asking, and I stopped saying it.

Instead, we talked about New York, about Dan and running, about what campground to stay at next—choosing to talk about what was light.

"You're doing really great with all this running, babe," I encouraged.

"Thanks," he said with a smile. "It's not too bad when there's someone else driving the car."

Dan was already parked and waiting somewhere up ahead. He'd given us a happy beep when he'd passed.

"I can't believe how close we are," Nate continued. "The start feels like a lifetime ago."

In all respects of the matter, it had been a lifetime ago—before days of driving, months of crewing, thousands of miles of running, multiple mechanical failures, a thieving photographer, countless predawn mornings, and perpetual nomadic living. It had been a lifetime, and it had only been five months. We were different people now that we had done this.

That afternoon, I crossed into West Virginia from East Steubenville across a wonderfully vintage yellow wooden bridge that spat me out onto a zippy highway paralleling the Ohio River. I ran along the winding throughway, and then onto quieter back roads for eight miles with Nate at my side before crossing into Pennsylvania. The jaunt across the tip of another state was just for fun—because I could.

By day, summer held fast to its stifling hot grip. But it was officially September now, and with it, glimmers of change and the relief that fall would bring poked through. Humidity receded at nightfall. Fresh mornings returned. A subtle hint of crisp nudged its way into the air. I felt it most acutely as I ran across the tip of West Virginia, with the leaves beginning their transition from their vibrant summer hues to pockets of slightly pale yellows and faint touches of the crimson that was to come.

For the next three days, I moved up and down thousands of feet of elevation—running, hiking, and leaning forward into the road. Then, over a ridge I'd go—coasting down, through and around with either Nate or Dan at my side. Unlike the vast, open, and brutally scorching miles of Iowa, Pennsylvania's roads were shaded and beautiful, bringing a sense of calm to the effort. There were breathtaking overlooks of rock and forest, steel bridges above drifting waterways, white-steepled churches clanging their bells.

Afterward, together, the three of us would go grocery shopping to pick out dinner. Dan would cook, I'd wash the dishes, and Nate would put them away.

Tucked into our beds at night, I'd feel a sense of peace, wishing it had always been like this—Nate with the support of another, and that other being someone like Dan, who was altogether optimistic, easy, and helpful. Like my parents, I wished for Dan to stay. But also like my parents, he had a business of his own to run. So on the morning of September 8, we gathered up his sparse belongings and dropped him at a bus station in Pittsburgh.

"I really appreciate your help," I said to him, embracing him in a tight hug. Not one thing this week had been a burden to him, not even when we'd booked him a bus ticket for the cheapest day of the week—and the ride would take him at least thirteen hours and include two transfer stops along the way. He'd arrive in Milwaukee just before midnight.

My appreciation for him was overwhelming.

"No problem at all," he said genuinely, holding me by my shoulders. "I'm happy to do it."

And I knew that he meant it.

Upon Dan's departure, Nate and I took no time to be alone, driving twenty-five minutes west to the Pittsburgh International Airport to pick up Steph.

"Hey!" I shouted to her as she walked out of the terminal wing.

She ambled down the gangway, carrying a large rectangular duffel bag and brimming backpack stuffed with enough items for an eleven-day stay with us in the RV. It was an immediate and stark contrast to Dan's meager supplies.

I went to her and threw my arms around her in a bear hug, nearly toppling her over. "You made it!"

"I am here to save your run!" She chuckled. It was a warm laugh I had come to know well. It matched her kind, crinkling eyes and tender demeanor. She was like a sister, and hugging her was home.

"Thanks for coming, Steph," Nate said, trailing behind me, arriving at her and giving her a hug as well. "I'm excited to show you around so you can see what the run is *really* like."

She laughed again. "Happy to be here," she said, clapping him on the shoulder. "Sounds like a fun challenge."

Before heading back toward the route, we decided to spend the day in Pittsburgh, eating ice cream and touring the waterways on a Just Ducky water boat tour. This was a vacation for Steph, after all. Graduating from college with a medical laboratory science degree, Steph started her career at a university hospital in Minnesota. She got herself a regular schedule, an apartment, a fancy gym membership, and began paying off her student loans. To come here, she'd had to submit a request for time off with her employer, which felt different to me than my parents and Dan shuffling their businesses around to accommodate a trip. I didn't appreciate one more than the other, but still, she had a set number of days each year, and she'd used a majority of them to help Nate crew me across Pennsylvania— rather than, say, using them instead to go to a beach vacation resort that served drinks with umbrellas and steak for dinner.

Crewing me was work, but I wanted it to be fun, so we purchased tickets for a duck boat tour, and then she and I sat side by side in the bench seats while Nate found a spot between me and an elderly woman with short hair and red bifocals. The duck boat engine roared to life, and we rumbled off into the water.

"Known as the City of Bridges," the tour guide said into a midgrade microphone that hummed and crackled over the motor and lapping waves. "Pittsburgh has 445 bridges in total that cross over the three rivers that converge here–the Allegheny, the Monongahela, and the Ohio. In fact," he said with pride, "we have more bridges here than they do in Venice!"

I leaned toward Steph. "Four hundred and forty-five!" I said, raising my eyebrows. "More than Venice."

She tilted her head toward me. "That's a lot of bridges."

"What'd you say?" Nate said, almost needing to yell over the motor, leaning my way.

"She was just saying that's a lot of bridges," I said, shouting back. He nodded.

We sat for a bit, each watching the skyline of Pittsburgh drift by–PNC Park, Heinz Stadium, the Carnegie Science Center. Steph snapped pictures with her phone.

"I'm really excited you're here," I said to Steph after she'd captured a photo. "I really appreciate you taking time off work and using it to help us."

She shrugged and gave me a smile. "I'm happy to be here. Gave me something to look forward to."

Steph had had a bit of a trying summer herself. Right about the time Nate had proposed to me on a mountain in California, Steph's partner of three years had cleared her things out of their shared apartment while Steph had been at work. I'd called to tell her that I was engaged, and she had told me Kim had left.

"You'll be surprised to know that I've been running a bit in preparation," she said.

"No way. Really?" I exclaimed. Steph was one hell of a soccer goalie, but as long as I had known her, running hadn't been her thing.

"Just a few miles here and there," she said. "Nothing big. But I figured if I was coming out to help, I should probably be able to run a little too."

"Well, I'll take it. Is that how you lost all the weight?"

She shook her head. "I haven't been eating much," she said, looking at me, and then out toward the water, "I've been doing a bit of smoking instead. I'm hoping this helps."

Steph looked like a shell of her former athletic self. Her T-shirt hung loosely off bony shoulders, and her face appeared sunken and thin. I had run the entire country and hadn't lost the weight she had. I didn't know what to say. There was nothing I could say. Steph was a serial monogamist and loyal companion. Kim's departure had been a huge blow to her fierce devotion—even if, maybe, it would end up for the better.

"Well, shoot. You know what? I can't say we have any menthol lights on board, but we could pick a pack up before our morning run if you'd like," I joked.

Steph gave me a deadpan look. I grinned and gave her a nudge. Nate leaned over. "Whatcha guys talking about?"

Steph leaned forward to meet his eye and said, "Nothing," while at the same time, I said, "Smoking."

Then she and I looked at each other and laughed at something neither of us could explain, folding into each other as we did.

CHAPTER TWENTY-ONE

Linger

I WAS IN NO rush to get to New York. It seemed all but a formality to have to run across Pennsylvania and New Jersey to prove that I was capable of it. The urgency that I had once used to attack the day all those months ago diminished in Milwaukee and gave way to a steeled confidence that nothing could stop me. If I had once melted because Nate had gotten lost, and I was exhausted and starving after seventeen miles; these things no longer fazed me.

Seventeen miles was simply a solid warm-up to the thirty that I would run, and I was just fine now with my hydration pack stuffed with snacks and money to buy whatever I needed at whatever business I came upon. My crossing plan had worked—dividing the country into thirds and continuing to build momentum as I ran. What had been a struggle then was now just a regular part of the day.

I had long since mastered blowing snot from my nose without a Kleenex and how to discreetly poop in a ditch. I'd run through pelting rain, whiteout snow, whipping winds, and the scorching sun. I had even taken care to see a doctor in Davenport, who'd looked at my porcelain bare feet with a furrowed brow.

"You ran here from California, and your feet look like this?" he'd asked.

They were the same pair I had always had, looking the same way they always had, flesh-colored toenails and all.

"Yeah," I'd replied, lifting my head from the exam table. The medical paper had crinkled. "This is what my feet look like."

He'd turned my feet about, and then shrugged. "Well, I had expected a few missing toenails and some bruising, to be honest. Maybe a few pesky blisters, at least. You know, I saw a guy last year doing this, and he could hardly walk," he said to me, gesturing toward my feet. "But you look perfectly healthy. I can't explain it. But I think you'll be just fine getting to New York."

He wasn't wrong. I was just fine. And now I was expected to arrive at my final destination by the end of the month on September 28, a date I'd chosen based on the 380 miles that remained.

It was difficult to take in.

In recent weeks, I'd tried to grasp the magnitude of what had happened and the distance I had run. Though not done yet, I was close enough to wonder about being done. I had physically run every mile and been present for it all. I was technically still doing it, but still, it was perplexing for me to gather up in my mind. This was something I had dreamed up less than two years ago in Barcelona, and I was now near completion. How had it all happened already? It felt like a dream. As I knew it would, it had gone by too fast.

Still, I set the date and spread the news. It had to be done. It would be over and not be returned to again, at least not in this way.

People began to ask me, "Would you ever run across America again?"

I would reply with a laugh. "Only for millions of dollars."

The adventure had been unbelievable, but raising the money was really all that mattered to me, and that was still a trickle.

Anyone following the endeavor, especially those traveling to New York for the finish, now knew that I expected to arrive on September 28. Plans for a celebration began to form.

Now, all I had to do was arrive.

"Home sweet home," I said to Steph, opening the door of the motorhome for her in the brightness of daylight. We had left the motorhome parked at a rural campground in West Virginia while we'd dropped off Dan and retrieved her, staying overnight in Pittsburgh after the ducky boat tour. The next morning, we'd driven back forty miles west to retrieve the vehicle, which was what we were doing now. We hadn't had time to move it forward before the crew exchange, and this was exactly the kind of back and forth that Nate had hated—and still did. He couldn't wait to be done and over with it, made obvious to everyone in the car because those were the stories he told.

"I can't tell you how many times I've had to drive back the full length of what Ashley's just run," he said, exasperated, telling his tales of the road. "You spend the whole day making progress, then *bam!* It's gone in less than an hour."

I left Steph in the motorhome's cabin to place her things in the nooks and crannies under the couch while I went to help Nate hitch the car in tow. We'd drive like this, hitched together for the day, assuming we could, with either Steph or Nate navigating the caravan after arriving at the route an hour from now. That was, until it was Steph's turn to drive—and she got lost.

Nate and I were out on the road along a rural highway near Wexford on a cloudy, sixty-degree morning when she called—her name and number flashing across my BlackBerry screen. I stopped to walk.

"Hey," I said, answering my phone. "What? You're lost?"

I listened while Nate threw out his hands and shook his head. I swatted at him.

"No, it's fine. You're parked, right?" I said, nodding. "Nope, it's fine. Just text me a pin of where you're at, and I'll take a look on my map."

She kept apologizing.

"Steph, it's fine. As long as nothing's damaged, it's fine."

Really, it was fine—kind of funny to me, actually, considering I had always thought of Steph as someone who could do anything. The fact that she'd gotten lost while being equipped with a smartphone navigation system was gold for our friendship. I'd have ammo for years to come.

"She's lost?" Nate said when I hung up.

"Apparently," I said, shaking my head and chuckling. I stared at my phone, waiting for her location pin.

"See," he said, like *I told you so*, gesturing with his hands. "People get lost on their first day. It's not as easy as you think."

I rolled my eyes–though he was right, I suppose. He'd gotten lost on his first day, and now so had she. I had been rather irritated with him at the time, and now, with Steph, it was fine. But the two were different. I was more relaxed now–well-trained and better equipped, having learned I needed to be.

"Well, lucky for her," I replied, "I've learned how to manage."

He gave me a nudge. I nudged him back. Then we both smiled and took off running to find Steph.

Steph, as it turns out, would end up being a horrible driver. She got lost, she got stuck, and much to my amazement, even with the help of GPS, she hardly knew which way was east. This was all very funny to me, just like my excessive consumption of peanut butter and mini-sized chocolate candies was funny to her. We sat together at a wooden picnic table four days into her stay, discussing these things.

"I mean, I just can't believe how much you eat," she said to me outside the camper at Black Moshannon State Park, a massive acreage of densely forested land in central Pennsylvania. It was deliciously shaded from the afternoon sun and exactly the kind of place where I'd set up camp and not depart from it for some time, if I had the option not to.

I'd made us each a heaping plate of food–mine a bit more heaping than hers–and brought them outside to where she lounged at the table.

"Well, I can't believe how *bad* you are at directions," I said, scooping a spoonful of instant wild rice into my mouth. "It's amazing, really."

"I do it for others," she said, joking. "I'd feel bad if I made everything look easy."

"I figured," I said, nodding. "You're so generous."

We sat quietly eating our food for a bit, shoveling grilled chicken, warm rice, and pita chips layered with globs of hummus into our mouths–replenishing what we'd burned over seventeen miles just hours earlier. We laughed about things that were happening and reminisced about things that had happened. Finally, I brought up her new interest.

"Have you heard from Lauren today?"

Steph shook her head. "Not yet. She's working. But I did send her a picture from the top of the RV this morning. I'm sure we'll talk later. Or not. Whatever."

Steph tried to act indifferent, shrugging and looking off into the woods like she was just enjoying the moment and not thinking about a girl she liked, but she wasn't. Steph had been introduced to Lauren recently through her roommate, and now they were "just talking." While Nate and I ran, Steph lazed upon the roof of the motorhome, sunning herself and texting a woman. Driving woes aside, it was turning out to be a pretty nice vacation for her after all.

"Whatcha doing?" Nate said, hopping out of the motorhome–freshly showered and with a plate full of food in his hand. The shocks of the vehicle squeaked as he descended the metal steps.

Steph shoved a pita chip in her mouth, and I got the distinct feeling that she wasn't talking about Lauren to much of anyone, except me and maybe one other friend.

"Oh, you know," I said, offering nothing. "Just catching up."

He nodded, sitting next to me at the table. Steph sat across from us. "All right then," he said, taking a bite of his chicken and rice. "When are you thinking we head back out?"

Eleven miles remained before I was done running for the day.

"We were thinking of going swimming first," I told him. The campground had a sandy freshwater beach just a short walking distance from our campsite. "The beach looks amazing. I was thinking we could do that, and then head back out around like four or so."

"*Tsk*. Why didn't you say something? I just showered."

"Well, I didn't know you were going to shower," I pointed out.

"I just figured it's not that hot out. I thought we'd head back out sooner and just be done for the day."

"Well..." I shrugged. "We want to go swimming."

Nate sat and looked at me, and then turned toward his plate. "It would have been nice if you had told me."

"I'm telling you now. Does that count?" I smiled.

He looked at me from the side of his eye, and then back at his plate.

I looked at Steph with big eyes, not fully grasping his irritation. What was there to do anyway? Be done earlier, and then do what, exactly? It was nice now, perfect for an afternoon swim.

"We won't be long," I said. "Just a quick little dip."

"Yeah," Steph said, nodding. "Definitely not long."

"Forget it," he said, standing up and taking his plate with him. "Just let me know when you two are done at the beach."

Down at the water, Steph and I laid out our towels side by side atop sand as fine as cinnamon sugar. The soft, warm granules squished between my bare toes, and the sun shone gently on my face through an opening in the trees.

I swam into the water, letting it wash my salty skin and cool my warm face. The beach was an inlet that traveled to a larger lake under a nearby bridge. That was the road I'd run across. Where we were, though, the water was shallow and warm, yet refreshing.

Wading into the shallows, I allowed myself to float upon the surface, my ears submerged and my eyes to the powder-blue sky. I saw the tops of trees, birds flying about, drifts of translucent clouds lazily floating by. At the parking lot, a young couple parked their car and began unloading a picnic. Fishermen towing their boat crossed the cement bridge.

Back on the towels, Steph lay flat on her belly, head to the side with her eyes shut. I walked from the water and did the same–lying myself flat on my belly too, resting my head to the side, closing my eyes.

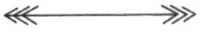

DAYS LATER, I HOOFED it up a steep stretch of road near what I hoped would be the top. I could never be sure until I'd summited and either saw what was generally *more* up, or saw a decline that would continue to go down, around the bends and turns, and then *more* down—until finally, the down would be as down as it would go, made obvious by the valley I'd arrived at, with a stretch of river rushing through its center. There, inevitably, would be an adorable little town nestled along the water. I'd run along its main street and head back up.

Up.

Up.

This was my path now, in the heart of the Appalachian Mountains, a stretch of ranges in the east that span from Canada to Alabama and were a mere hundred-and-eighty-some miles from my finish.

I knew of the Appalachians, though not in the way I knew of the Rockies. They weren't a collection of ridges and peaks majestically soaring above the tree line. Rather, they were tree-covered and rolling—making it difficult to pin their tops when traveling among their foliage, but a mountain range all the same, with a long trail in the center that followed ridges from north to south.

The famous Appalachian Trail was the first I knew of its kind, where the distance was so long that people took extended periods of time to hike it, the thought of which captured me—to pack up one's things and stuff them in a bag to be carried on one's back in the woods for weeks on end.

I had been five, and fully, unabashedly myself when I'd learned that people did this. Independent and forward, it was these qualities of mine that had brought me to know about the mountains in the first place.

"Want to know why my dad rearranged the office?" I'd blurted out knowingly to his assistant, Ray, a middle-aged associate who'd seemed to be nerdy and quiet.

The adults in the room—my father, mother, and Ray—had all stopped talking and looked at me.

I'd continued. "It's because he wanted to see your computer screen to make sure that you're working."

I had overheard my parents talking about this very thing some nights before in the kitchen—that my father had his concerns about how Ray was using his time, that he had spent the day rearranging the office so he could watch Ray. I'd sat on the carpet in the next room with my siblings watching TV, but had been listening to my parents talk instead, not understanding why my father wouldn't just say something to Ray's face–thinking that if Ray knew, he'd be able to do better.

So, one afternoon shortly thereafter, I raced into my father's office and announced to Ray the very thing that he should know. And though I don't recall the moments after, I can only assume it was the kind of uncomfortable that takes weeks, if ever, to recover from.

What I do remember was that later, at home, my parents had gently explained to me that some things we don't say. Some things hurt people's feelings. As they'd spoken, a pressure had filled my chest. I'd been devastated.

I hurt Ray? How?

I only thought that *I* would want to know, so *he* might want to know. For some time, I carried Ray's hurt around with me, trying to make up for it every week by asking my father how he was doing. One time, instead of saying "Fine," he'd replied, "He's good. He took a long vacation this summer. He's hiking the Appalachians."

Twenty-one years later, I was in the Appalachians too, telling Steph that same story and laughing at my brash innocence as we crested another sharp incline near the end of another thirty-some-mile day.

"You would say something like that," she said, shaking her head. "You've hardly changed."

"Whatever," I replied, *thwacking* her arm, walking at her side. "I've changed."

She paused. "Yeah, I know," she said sentimentally. "You have changed."

I looked at her, knowing we were no longer talking about my filter, or lack thereof, and smiled back. "Thanks." Then, a few moments later, I said, "But not *that* much, right?"

"No, of course not," she said, shaking her head, encouraging. "Not that much."

We continued hiking. Instead of resting for the afternoon, Nate, she, and I had decided to take an hour-long lunch and keep moving. The days on the road had been long recently, but they had been beautiful. I was running more now than I had been in past months—twenty-eight miles, thirty miles, thirty-four miles in one day, moving under the canopy of dense maples that changed their colors while the sun shone brightly, and lush service berries filled the peripheral.

It helped, too, that the weather had cooled—the air settling around a pleasant sixty-five degrees at high noon. And without the RV at a campground, I found no reason to lounge around like we had at Black Moshannon. The past two nights we'd stayed on the road, sleeping in a Walmart parking lot, and then at a service station with overnight parking.

It was late in the afternoon now, and parked about a mile or so away somewhere up ahead was Nate with the vehicles. We'd find him and then look for another free place to camp.

At the top of the hill, a roadside eatery with a charming outdoor patio appeared.

"Oh!" I said of the bar and grill at the same time that Steph said, "Cute!"

"Wanna stop for a drink?" I asked, looking at her.

"You bet I do," she replied.

Sitting in a weathered plastic chair, I chopped the ice of my double Captain and Coke with a black straw and then took a long pull. A wave of spiced rum and liquid sugar tingled my throat. My blood warmed.

Steph poked at her phone.

I watched the grass, the trees, the road, seeing an occasional car zoom by. I thought how curious it was that I was sitting here doing this with Steph, that I'd never be sitting here doing this with her again.

"So what's next, you think?" she said at last. "You really going to do this relay thing?"

"For sure!" I said without thinking, surfacing from my thoughts. "I mean, I'll try. It really depends on whether people sign up."

Despite the fact that Nate and I continued to differ on this topic, I pressed on with the idea, though more subtly and thoughtfully than before, more or less dancing around it in his presence. I continued to meet runners who wanted to do something like I was doing right now—but didn't have the time or the resources to do it. And I was continually asked, like Steph was asking me now, what was next. To that point, either I meant to raise half a million dollars for the cause or I did not. Either I was running to fund research, or I wasn't. For me, I already knew what was true.

She looked out at the road and then back at me. "Now that I've been out here, I can totally see it. But I definitely couldn't imagine it when you first told me."

"Runners'll get it," I told her. "People do destination races all the time. They plan their whole year around them. If we provide the motorhome and the crew, and all they have to do is fundraise and show up, well, then..." I shrugged, like it was obvious that I'd fill a relay team of people wanting to run across America.

"So you're providing the crew?" she challenged me.

I flicked my straw at her.

"Details," I replied, dodging the question, knowing she knew that I wanted to crew. "I'll figure that out when the time comes."

Just then, my phone buzzed with a text.

Are you close? the message from Nate said.

I made a face.

"What?" Steph asked.

"Uh." I paused. "I forgot to text Nate that we were stopping. He just asked where we were."

She glanced to the side, and then picked up her drink and started chugging. I picked up my drink, too, and did the same. Then we gathered our things and hurried our asses up the road.

"Why didn't you text me?" He laid in when we arrived. "I had no idea where you were. Why are you even *drinking* right now?"

"It was *a* drink, Nate. And I'm sorry," I said defensively. "It wasn't planned. We just saw the place and decided to stop, and then we were talking, and I forgot to text. Okay? It's not a big deal."

Steph slipped past us into the motorhome, gently closing the door behind her.

"A big deal? You're on the road. I didn't know where you were!" he said, his voice rising. "I'm sitting here for an hour thinking who knows what, and instead, you're off having a drink with your mate!"

"An hour? Come on," I said, rolling my eyes, raising my voice too. "It was like thirty minutes. And you know what? I'm *fine*. I've made it twenty-six years without you. I don't need you to watch over me."

"Thanks," he said, visibly hurt and angrier by the moment. "Thanks a whole lot. I'm out here trying to help, and you're off just doing whatever the hell you want."

I wanted to scream. I wasn't doing whatever the hell I wanted. I was doing exactly as I should–running more miles than I needed to, coordinating my finish, and trying to enjoy the last bit of what remained of this unbelievably incredible experience–which he was welcome to join.

I wanted to yell at him for being so uptight, for wanting this to be over, for sucking the fun out of what remained by pining for the end, like what we were doing right now wasn't good enough. Whatever his problem was wasn't mine. He was unhappy. That was clear. But fixing that wasn't up to me.

Some things we don't say. Some things hurt people's feelings.

Instead, I took the pack I held in my hand, light with water from what remained in the bladder, and started walking.

"Ashley! What are you doing?" he called after me.

I swung the pack around my back and put my arms through the straps. "What does it *look* like I'm doing?" I said over my shoulder.

And at that, I ran.

Sometime later, after the sun had gone, I heard the car approach behind me, slowing at my side. The headlights cast a soft glow upon the road.

He had already come after me once in the motorhome, Steph somewhere inside the cabin, and instead of looking his way, I'd steeled my eyes to the road ahead.

Don't even fucking try to talk to me, my face had said.

He'd idled the beast at my side for a moment and then driven on.

Now, with the motorhome parked somewhere safe, I presumed, they tried again in the car.

Steph called to me softly from the open passenger window. "Hey."

"Hey," I said, slowing to a walk.

"What'd ya think?" she asked.

"Where are we at?" I said back, not knowing exactly how far I had run, only knowing it had felt like an hour or so, and now it was dark.

"You're at forty-four miles for the day," Nate said, leaning forward to see me. The dome light brightened the interior of the car, and I could see his face—no longer hurt and angry. Rather, he was trying earnestly to get me off the road.

I looked up ahead. I was tired—body and mind. The swearing in my mind had gone silent sometime back, leaving only the sound of shoes gripping concrete and lungs breathing air. It's when I knew I could be done, when all I heard was my body in a run.

"All right," I replied, turning toward the car. "We can stop."

I climbed into the back seat and looked out the window. Nate maneuvered us around with a Y-turn to drive back the way we had come. We drove in silence, listening to a mixed CD—Steph texting, Nate driving, me looking out the window—until we arrived at the RV, which was parked on the side of the road in a wide, flat pullout. Inside, I went straight to the fridge and started pulling out piles of food—turkey lunch meat, a block of cheddar cheese, a jar of pickles.

"I made you vegetables," Nate said, coming in last, standing near the captain's chair closest to the door. "But she ate them."

I turned from the fridge to look at him, and then to Steph, who was sitting at the dinette table behind me.

"What?" I asked, confused.

"I made you vegetables," he said again, explaining to both of us. "They were delicious. I really wanted you to try them. But she ate them when you and I were outside before you took off running."

I looked at Steph for clarification.

"I was hungry." She shrugged. "They *were* really good," she added.

I looked back at Nate. "We can make other ones," I said, not caring much about vegetables I couldn't have anyway.

"I made *those* ones," he yelled, hitting the back of the chair with an open hand. "For *you*."

Then he stormed out of the RV and slammed the door behind him.

I stared at the door for a long moment. Then I turned to Steph. "It's not about the vegetables," I said.

"I know," she replied. "I know."

CHAPTER TWENTY-TWO

Searching Middle

SIGNIFICANCE LAY IN HOW insignificant it felt to cross the George Washington Bridge into New York City on the final day of my run across America. Standing on the west side of the bridge in New Jersey, just a mere thirteen miles remained between me and the conclusion of my journey.

At the New York City Hall where I was headed, Montel Williams stood beside my mother and the Mayor atop a cascade of steps covered with media, cause officials, supporters, and friends and family who had flown into New York from around the country to be there. They all waited for me to arrive, to triumphantly complete my 3,288-mile run across America—an endurance challenge of such magnitude physically, financially, and emotionally that only a select few would ever attempt the feat, and even fewer would actually finish.

Thirteen miles from this achievement, I ran across the bridge into New York on a dull and sunless Tuesday with a quaint group of men from a local running club—and Nate along on a bike. We crossed the state line in clumsy silence—me, not knowing what to say for this special occasion to these men I had just met, and them trailing behind me just a step, giving me the space we all assumed I needed to absorb the moment.

The date was September 28, exactly 190 days from the morning I had crossed the Golden Gate Bridge to start the journey, and the overcast clouds that matched the concrete sidewalk hid the New York City skyline behind a mass of dense fog. I looked at the cumulation of gray through a chain-link fence high atop a pathway above the Hudson River and waited to feel something profound.

It eluded me.

Is this it?

To get here, I had run twenty-four miles a day, six days a week, for six months, becoming the sixteenth woman to ever run across the country. I'd burned an estimated 300,000 calories, run through eleven pairs of running shoes, crossed thirteen states, traversed three mountain ranges, lost eighteen pounds, and managed to endure only two blisters and one bout of heat exhaustion as the extent of my injuries. Surely, a surge of emotion would overcome me.

The suspension bridge swayed with a stream of steady traffic. Water waves I couldn't hear below me lapped against the shoreline. Bikers from behind called, and we moved to make room.

At the east end of the bridge, I headed south.

I counted the donations, a touch over $56,000 in fundraising for MS research, and felt disappointed. Need I run all the way across the entire country for money I could have raised at a well-promoted charity event back home?

It had been an ambitious commitment in the first place. No one had set the goal for me, and no one would blame me if I fell short. Yet, still. It lingered, like a promise I'd made to myself despite what anyone else had to say. It was the value I'd given the whole damn effort. It was a sum that I'd thought could make a difference—for my mom, for others, for me. The enormity of my athletic achievement felt hollow without it.

The answer was yet to come.

Like a seed planted in the spring, a mission grew deep and wide over the 190 days I ran from west to east, nurtured by runners like me wanting to use the power of their running for a purpose greater than themselves.

SEARCHING MIDDLE

I'd thought I had been called to run across America for MS. But that was incomplete. I had been called to run across America for MS and lead others to do the same. My experience was a gift, not of my own making. I felt a push to pass it on.

In the months and years that followed, instead of it being a finish, New York would emerge as a middle. A weird, vague, searching middle where I would find that the truest test of my endurance lay far beyond my New York finish.

It showed itself in the quiet unraveling of my relationship with Nate. We tried—I followed him to Australia for a bit, and we settled into a more typical life. And still, my commitment to the nonprofit pulled at me like a vortex. One that took my entire focus, time, and energy—and I was glad to let it. Once given some space, we would discover that we were both kind people, not made for each other. And with time, that would be okay.

It revealed itself in the constant tug-of-war between my desire for stability and the uncertain, relentless work of building a charity event unlike anything else.

It was unknown to me then, as I ran those thirteen miles to the steps at New York's city hall, feeling a mix of pride and disappointment, that this was the beginning of something much bigger—that I would lead a motley crew of runners from all across the country in an event that would be the only of its kind—America's first 3,260-mile ultra relay run.

The runners would do for one week what I had done for six months—run a marathon a day for six consecutive days until they arrived at their finish 160 miles later, where they'd hand off the baton to their teammate, who would do the same. End to end, twenty-one runners lined up. Five months later, our final runner would bring the team to its finish in New York. To participate, they'd each raised at least $10,000 to be there, with many surpassing that goal. And so would others I'd find, as the event continued each year thereafter to involve hundreds of runners, thousands of donors, and bring millions of dollars toward the cause.

To rely on myself to run across America was one thing—maybe even a simple thing for someone as fiercely independent as I was.

But to depend on others, and to learn to trust that I could—that cracked me open and began to heal what MS took in the first place. Runners showed up and stayed, through years of building the charity, and revealed to me the community that we were always meant to have.

It would come to me then, the well of emotion I'd expected at my finish in New York City, on the opposite side of the country—in California, as my first relay runner prepared to start the charity's inaugural event. After the banners were lifted and the interviews taped and my runner tightened up their laces one last time—a rise of appreciation rushing from within my body with such force that I folded into myself, crying deep, unreserved tears. The kind that comes from immense gratitude, having lived such experiences since that morning in Barcelona, where my twenty-four-year-old self ran three miles upon a treadmill, whimsically wishing up a journey that became far less than the one that I would actually travel.

What a gift it was, the life that unfolded because I dared to begin.

NOTES

To learn more about the nonprofit I founded, MS Run the US, visit the charity's website at http://msruntheus.org. The organization has grown and expanded since my journey in 2010, with a dedicated mission to raising awareness and funds for those living with multiple sclerosis (MS)–to provide hope and resources for well-being, to aid those living with disability from the disease, and to support research to stop it.

You can find me on my website to connect or follow my journey at http://ashleymschneider.com.

My mother died of complications from MS in 2017, though she was able to witness many years of the charity's growth and take part in its events–always at the heart of its mission and values. If I could change one thing about her life with MS, it would be a more focused, consistent effort to support her health through nutrition and lifestyle modifications. An anti-inflammatory diet, daily movement, and even something as simple as intentional breathing are gentle but powerful tools–backed by research–to help reduce inflammation and improve quality of life for everyone, but especially important for those living with MS. I often wonder how different her life might have been with those adjustments in place.

Montel Williams supported me from the very beginning, when I first reached out to him in 2009. From day one, he's been quick to respond, generous with his platform, and genuinely committed to elevating both my story and the mission of MS Run the US.

I'm deeply grateful that he took a chance on me and this idea. His support extended beyond my 2010 run across America—he championed the nonprofit through its early years, helping to build the relay's visibility through partnerships and media spotlights.

One of the key individuals who played a significant role in my 2010 run across America is represented in this book under a changed name—Nate. While I've chosen not to use his real name for legal and privacy reasons, I am deeply grateful to him for his willingness to take on this adventure with me and for staying at my side at such a formative time. His intention and care were instrumental as the run evolved and as the foundation of MS Run the US began to take shape.

The quote at the beginning of this book is a favorite of mine, clipped from a women's soccer magazine when I was twelve. It has traveled with me ever since, always within view. Each day it reminds me that I have the power to create my own greatness—I need only to work hard for it.

The poem referenced by my father in chapter 20:

"Don't Quit" by John Greenleaf Whittier

When things go wrong, as they sometimes will,
When the road you're trudging seems all uphill.
When the funds are low and the debts are high,
And you want to smile, but you have to sigh.
When care is pressing you down a bit,
Rest, if you must, but don't you quit.

Life is strange with its twists and turns
As every one of us sometimes learns.
And many a failure comes about
When he might have won had he stuck it out.
Don't give up though the pace seems slow—
You may succeed with another blow.

NOTES

Success is failure turned inside out—
The silver tint of the clouds of doubt,
And you never can tell how close you are,
It may be near when it seems so far;
So stick to the fight when you're hardest hit
It's when things seem worst that you must not quit.

For all the sad words of tongue or pen
The saddest are these: "It might have been!"

ACKNOWLEDGMENTS

"Thank you" is such a common expression that I hesitate to use it here as it hardly captures the depth of gratitude I feel for those who have kept me moving forward—toward writing and publishing this book.

To my husband, Aaron, and our children—Primrose, Sierra, and AJ—my deepest thanks for encouraging my dreams, for accepting me as I am, for cheering me on when the work felt hard and overwhelming, and for providing me a safe and loving place to rest.

To my parents: Thank you for the experiences you gifted me before you passed. I am who I am because you nurtured me to be so. Your love and support were uniquely yours, and I'm one lucky kid to have been yours.

To those who wish to remain anonymous—who were early supporters of my nonprofit and continued to give me hope when I did not always see the light—I am indebted to you for seeing in me what I could not always see in myself. Your unwavering belief in the power of my story is a cornerstone of what I have been able to achieve.

I wrote the majority of this book in my basement over the course of four years while my children ran around upstairs being tended to by a sitter or my husband. A critical turning point in my writing and how the story was structured came during a three-day writing escape, when I was gifted the opportunity to tuck myself away from the world in a cabin up north in Wisconsin. Randy and Laura, thank you for your support of my work and your willingness to open your hearts and your home to me, untethered by expectations. The world needs more people like you.

Some people enter your life with such presence and energy that it's almost unnerving. Meeting Robin Arzón in 2012–before her rise on social media and her reign as the Queen of Peloton–was like that. Robin was a powerful presence long before the public recognition, and her example has mentored me in ways she may never fully know. Robin, your intelligence, ferocity, and challenge to others to rise to their best selves have both frustrated and empowered me–always in the best ways. Thank you for shining unapologetically, for showing up as you are, and for encouraging others to do the same. I am deeply honored by your words and profoundly grateful that you contributed the foreword to this book.

I was able to write a book of this magnitude because of the editors who offered sharp, honest feedback on pacing, story arc, and clarity. Amanda Gersh, your mentorship transformed the way I write. Thank you for pulling the best from me and for always being so much fun to work with. Katie Wilson, you are a writing genius. I am endlessly grateful for the times you showed up–often on short notice–with insight, elegance, and grace.

To my siblings–April, Aaron, and Dawn ("D" for done): thanks for being the best crew to grow up with. Our memories are many, and our stories are still unfolding. I wouldn't trade us for the world.

To my girlfriends: I still can't believe I have friendships like ours–full of love, laughter, truth, and support. Thank you for teaching me how to trust, for embracing the messiness and realness of life by my side, and for giving me the confidence to share this story with the world. Your love carries me.

I started my nonprofit in 2009, more or less out of a logistic necessity for my endeavor, and continued to show up for its growth because of the people who arrived and affirmed its place in the running and MS communities. It exists today because of those that came after me–the runners, my staff, the longtime donors, the volunteers, and its supporters. This would be a terribly lonely road without you. For your support and effort, I am thankful beyond measure and honor what we have built–together.

ABOUT THE AUTHOR

Ashley M. Schneider is the founder of MS Run the US Inc., a nonprofit inspired by her 3,288-mile run across America to raise awareness for multiple sclerosis in honor of her mother. Under her leadership, the organization has mobilized hundreds of runners, thousands of supporters, and raised over $4 million for MS research and direct financial aid—becoming a powerful force in MS awareness, research, and community support. A sought-after speaker and writer, Ashley shares powerful stories about beginnings, persistence, and transforming pain into purpose. She lives near Milwaukee, Wisconsin, with her husband and three children.

www.ingramcontent.com/pod-product-compliance
Lightning Source LLC
Chambersburg PA
CBHW020241010526
44107CB00039B/1454/J